Toxic Mold

Your Quick-Start Guide to Spot, Stop, and Recover From Mold Exposure

Essential Facts and First Steps to Tackle Mold Fast

Yvette Farkas

Copyright:

Toxic Mold: Your Quick-Start Guide to Spot, Stop, and
Recover From Mold Exposure
Essential Facts and First Steps to Tackle Mold Fast
© 2025 by Yvette Farkas

ISBN:
Paperback: 978-1-998333-23-3
Hardcover: 978-1-998333-25-7
E-book: 978-1-998333-24-0

Published by:
Singing Soul Books
Website: www.singingsoulbooks.com
Email: info@singingsoulbooks.com

Disclaimer:
The information, techniques, and resources in this book are
intended to educate readers about mold exposure, prevention,
and recovery. While every effort has been made to ensure the
accuracy and reliability of the content, the author and publisher
are not medical professionals and assume no responsibility for
any health outcomes, damages, or losses resulting from the
use of the suggestions provided. Readers are encouraged to
consult mold-literate health practitioners, environmental
experts, or other relevant professionals before applying any

methods, especially if they have existing health conditions or concerns. Mold exposure and recovery are highly individual experiences, and results may vary based on personal circumstances, environmental factors, and application.

The author and publisher disclaim any liability, loss, or risk incurred directly or indirectly from the use of this book's content. Readers are solely responsible for their own decisions, actions, and outcomes related to mold management and health recovery. This guide is a starting point, not a definitive solution, and we encourage you to seek additional expert guidance or resources as needed to support your journey. By reading this book, you agree that the author and publisher are not liable for any adverse consequences arising from its use.

Approach your mold recovery with care, awareness, and professional support—this book is your companion, not a prescription.

Table of Contents

Introduction

Many people clearly remember when they first noticed it—those seemingly harmless black spots on the wallpaper, on the window sill in the kitchen, or that musty smell that permeated the basement and bathroom. They wrote it off as "just a little mold," as most people do, but as their health began to deteriorate inexplicably—unrelenting fatigue that was unabated by caffeine, unexplained rashes that refused to go away, and persistent brain fog that made even simple tasks difficult—they realized they were grappling with something far more sinister.

The real culprit—toxic mold—came to light after years of incorrect diagnoses, expensive and unsuccessful therapies, and numerous hours spent researching their symptoms. Mold isn't just an eyesore—it's a silent invader that can wreak havoc on your health and home, often without you even realizing it.

This guide represents more than just the journey of countless individuals; it embodies the collective wisdom of hundreds of survivors, medical professionals, and environmental experts who have dedicated themselves to understanding and combating mold-related illness.

If you're reading this, it's likely that you or someone you care about is dealing with mysterious health problems or living or working in a moldy environment. Perhaps you have recurrent sinus issues, anxiety, allergies, or chronic exhaustion. Maybe there's a musty smell in your house that you can't seem to get rid of, or your kids have ongoing respiratory problems. Mycotoxins and toxic mold could be a hidden reason.

> **Myth:**
> Black mold is the only dangerous kind.
>
> **Fact:**
> Many molds can produce mycotoxins, and color doesn't determine danger; green, white, or even hidden molds can harm your health too.

Imagine a home where you, your loved ones—parents, partners, kids, even pets—feel vibrant and well. The steps you take today to tackle mold can make that a reality. Let's create a space that nurtures everyone's well-being, from the ground up. Discover simple ways to keep mold at bay and watch your family thrive in a cleaner, fresher environment. Your journey to a healthier, happier home starts here.

What Is Mold?

- **Definition**: A type of fungi that reproduces through microscopic spores

- **Growth Requirements**:

  - Moisture (key factor)

  - Food source (organic materials)

  - Appropriate temperature (usually 40-100°F/4.4-37.8°C.)

  - Time (can begin growing within 24-48 hours)

- **Spread**: Through air currents, water, or physical contact

Understanding Fungi, Mold, and Mycotoxins

- **Fungi**: Related to algae, consisting of mycelium networks. They feed on dead plant or animal remains, not sunlight or air. Fungi play essential roles in ecosystems as decomposers.

- **Mold**: A type of fungus that thrives in damp or humid environments. It can grow on various surfaces like wood, walls, or food.

- **Non-Toxic Molds**: These don't produce mycotoxins but can still cause allergy-like symptoms such as sneezing, coughing, or skin irritation.

- **Toxic Molds**: Specific types that produce mycotoxins, leading to potentially serious health issues.

Mycotoxins Explained

- **What They Are**:

  - Natural toxic compounds produced by certain molds

  - Invisible to the naked eye

  - Can persist even after mold is dead

- **Common Types**:

  - **Aflatoxins**

    - Produced by Aspergillus species

    - Often found in stored grains

    - Known carcinogen

  - **Ochratoxins**

    - Found in coffee, wine, and cereals

    - Can cause kidney damage

  - **Trichothecenes**

    - Produced by black mold

    - Highly immunosuppressive

    - Can cause neurological symptoms

Types of Toxic Mold

1. Stachybotrys (Black Mold)

- **Appearance**: Dark green or black
- **Common Locations**:
    - Water-damaged buildings
    - Paper products
    - Wood materials
- **Health Effects**:
    - Respiratory problems
    - Headaches
    - Memory loss
    - Nose bleeds

2. Aspergillus

- **Varieties**: Over 185 species
- **Common Locations**:
    - Air conditioning systems
    - Stored foods
    - House dust
- **Health Effects**:
    - Allergic reactions

- Lung infections

- Sinus infections

3. Penicillium

- **Appearance**: Blue-green

Tip:
Wear a mask—
mold spores hit
your lungs fast!

- **Common Locations**:

  - Wallpaper

  - Carpeting

  - Insulation

- **Health Effects**:

  - Chronic sinusitis

  - Bronchitis

  - Allergic reactions

Other Common Toxic Molds

- **Aspergillus flavus**: Found in damp walls, wallpaper, and stored food products

- **Aspergillus fumigatus**: Common airborne mold, prevalent indoors and outdoors

- **Aspergillus versicolor**: Grows in air conditioning and carpeting

- **Alternaria**: Grows on wood, drywall, or paint, causing severe respiratory symptoms

Mold Basics: What You Need to Know

- **Mold has a smell, but its mycotoxins don't**—You might smell something musty, but mycotoxins—the harmful parts of mold—have no smell. They can make your air toxic without you knowing.

- **Mold can affect your digestion**—It can grow in your intestines, stealing nutrients, triggering cravings, and causing bad breath or indigestion.

- **It's tied to allergies and sensitivities**—Mold can trigger allergies, food intolerances, and even make you more sensitive to chemicals or disharmonious electromagnetic fields.

- **Dust and moisture feed mold**—House dust, combined with dampness, helps mold grow, so dusting in hard-to-reach spots regularly is important.

- **Mold lives inside your home**—It likes to eat building materials like drywall, plywood, and cardboard. It can hide inside walls, ceilings, and floors.

- **Most Mold Stays Invisible**—It's so tiny you can't see it at first. By the time you spot black or green patches, it's already spread far.

- **Mold releases toxic gases**—These gases can contribute to "sick home syndrome" and various long-term health issues.

- **Water is mold's best friend**—Leaks, spills, or humidity give mold the perfect conditions to thrive.

- **Pets Feel Mold Too**—Your dog or cat might sneeze or act strange because mold hurts them too.

- **Mold Grows Quietly**—It can start growing in hours if it's wet or damp. It sneaks up, harming your home and health over time.

- **New Homes Aren't Safe**—Even brand-new homes can have mold from construction dust or trapped dampness, no matter how nice they look.

- **Mold Can Confuse Your Mind**—Feeling foggy or unable to think clearly? Mold might be affecting your brain.

- **Mold Likes Your Things**—It grows on damp books, rugs, or inside and on kids' toys, turning your belongings into hidden health risks.

Myth:
Mold on cheese means it's spoiled—throw it out.

Fact:
Blue cheeses like Roquefort use safe, intentional molds and are fine to eat, but if mold hits cheddar, cut an inch around hard types to save it—soft cheeses like Brie or mozzarella must get tossed since unseen spores spread fast.

Quick Wins: 10 Things You Can Do Today

Beat mold fast with these simple moves—no experts or big budgets needed.

1. **Ventilate Your Space**: Open windows for 15 minutes to cut humidity—mold hates fresh air.

2. **Spot Leaks:** Check under sinks and around pipes for drips; wipe dry with a towel.

3. **Dry Damp Spots:** Run a fan on wet carpets or walls for 10 minutes—stops mold's foothold.

4. **Kill Surface Mold:** Spray vinegar on shower grout, wait 1 hour, scrub—kills 82% of mold.

5. **Clean a Mold Zone:** Wipe fridge drip pans and seals with 3% hydrogen peroxide—mold's sneak attack foiled.

6. **Boost with Bioflavonoids:** Drink freshly squeezed lemon water and add lemon zest—bioflavonoids fight mycotoxins early.

7. **Bind Toxins:** Sprinkle 2 tbsp flax seeds on lunch—traps mycotoxins in your gut.

8. **Check Toys**: Soak kids' bath toys in vinegar for 15 minutes—stops hidden mold cold.

9. **Wash Pet Bowls:** Scrub pet water bowls with 3% hydrogen peroxide—keeps mold off their drink.

10. **Dry Pet Beds:** Shake out pet bedding, air dry in sun—mold hates a dry nap spot.

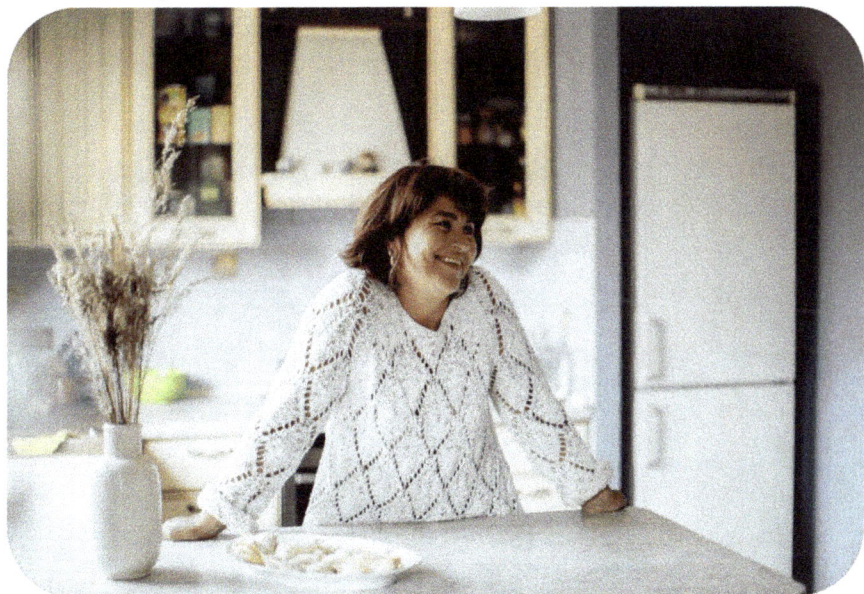

Mold-Killing Products at a Glance: What Works Best

Selecting a mold-killing method is like picking the right tool for the job—each has unique strengths. Knowing their effectiveness empowers you to tackle mold confidently. For severe infestations, call in professionals. For minor cases, consider these options. For a detailed explanation of how each of these works, with examples, go to the section titled "Mold-Cleaning Solutions: Efficacy, Uses, Safety."

- **UV-C Lighting** (254 nm, Ozone-Free): Kills 99%+ on exposed surfaces (EPA-backed), but doesn't penetrate. Ideal for air or surface sanitizing.

- **Hydrogen Peroxide** (3%): Kills up to 90% on contact, strong for deeper cleaning.

- **White Vinegar** (5-8%): Kills 82% on surface mold, best for light, non-porous spots.

- **Natural Solutions:** Varies—Benefect (thymol) nears 99% on surfaces; thyme, oregano, clove, cinnamon, eucalyptus, and tea tree essential oils hit 70-95% for mild cases.

- **Professional cleaners** (e.g., BenzaRid): Kills 95-99.99%, lab-tested, often hospital-grade for tough jobs.

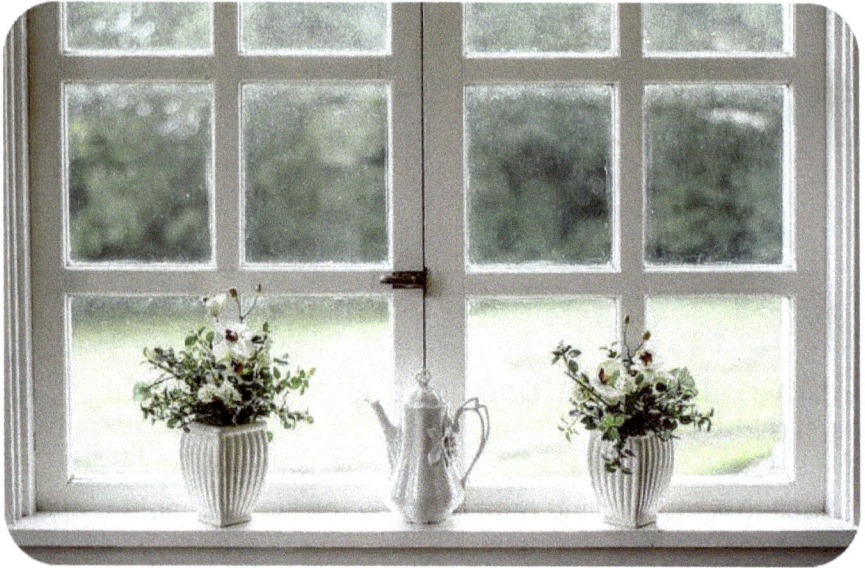

The Science of Exposure

How Exposure Occurs

- **Inhalation**

    - Most common route

    - Spores enter through nose/mouth

    - Can penetrate deep into lungs

- **Skin Contact**

    - Direct contact with moldy surfaces

    - Through contaminated water

    - Via airborne spores

- **Ingestion**

    - Contaminated food

    - Hand-to-mouth transfer

    - Contaminated water

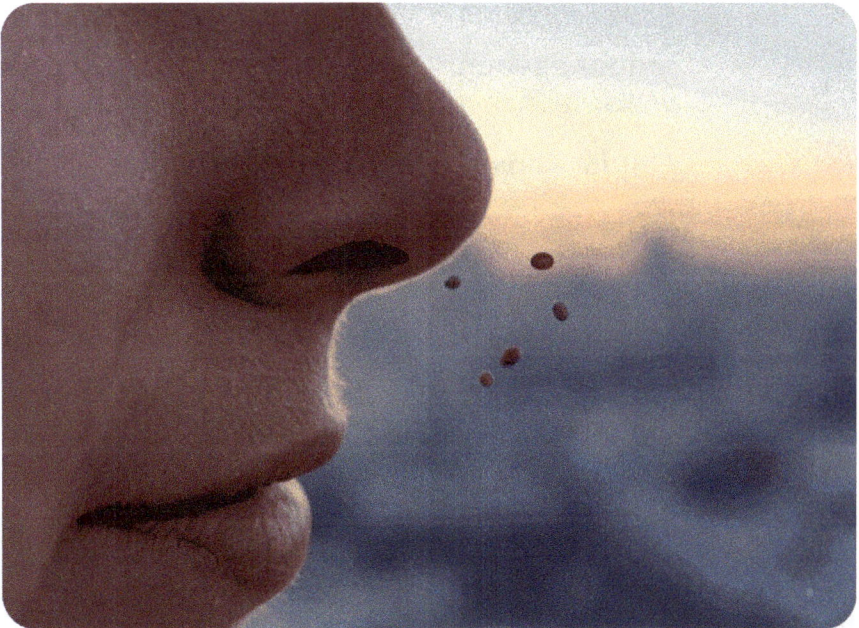

How Mycotoxins Harm Your Body

- **How They Enter**

  - **Airborne**: Enter through the respiratory tract, causing asthma, allergies, and sinus infections

  - **Leaky Gut**: Pass through the intestinal wall, affecting organs and skin

  - **Mitochondrial Disruption**: Can cause chronic fatigue, weakness, and oxidative stress

- **Sources of Mycotoxins**

  - **Contaminated food and feed** (especially grains, nuts, spices, coffee beans, dried fruits)

  - **Indoor environments with mold growth** (damp walls, ceilings, HVAC systems, bathrooms)

  - **Outdoor environments** (crops, soil)

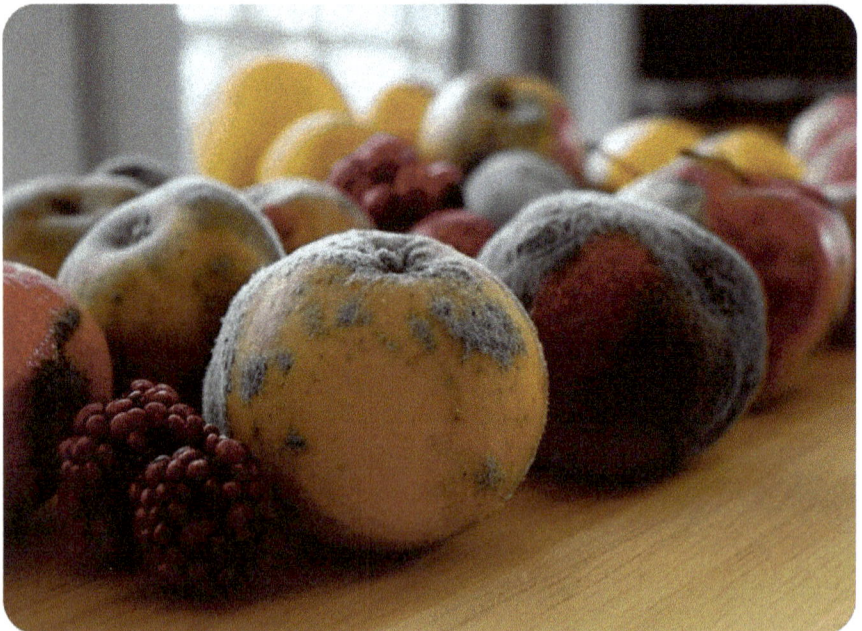

Symptoms of Mold Exposure

Non-Toxic Mold Symptoms

- Itchy Throat
- Cough
- Headache
- Eye Irritation
- Sinus Congestion
- Breathing Difficulties

Toxic Mold Symptoms

- Unexplained Weight Changes
- Mood Changes
- Numbness and Tingling
- Vertigo
- Cognitive Difficulties (Brain Fog, Poor Memory)
- Muscle Pain
- Tinnitus (Ringing in Ears)
- Digestive Issues
- Significant Fatigue
- Metallic Taste in Mouth
- Excessive Thirst
- Hormone Imbalance Symptoms

Who Is Affected by Mold?

Everyone is at Risk: Mold doesn't discriminate. Infants, the elderly, and everyone in between can be affected by mold exposure.

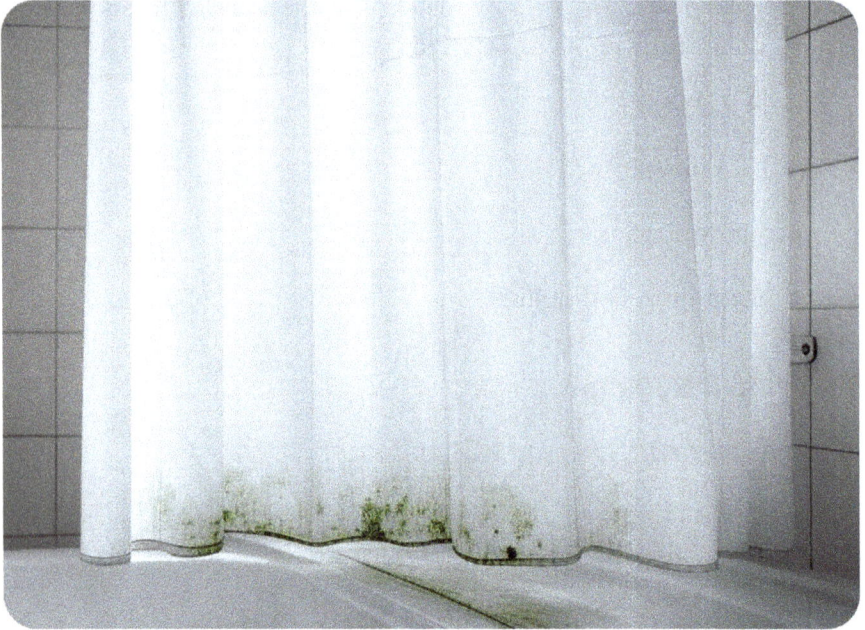

Health Impact on Humans

Symptoms of Mold Exposure in Humans

Exposure to mold can cause a wide range of symptoms, varying in severity depending on the level of exposure and individual susceptibility. If you're experiencing any of these symptoms, you may be suffering from mold exposure.

Respiratory Symptoms

- **Coughing**: Persistent cough that may be dry or productive

- **Wheezing**: A whistling sound when breathing, indicating airway constriction

- **Shortness of Breath**: Difficulty breathing, especially during physical activity

- **Nasal Congestion**: Stuffy or runny nose

- **Throat Irritation**: Sore throat or a feeling of irritation in the throat

Allergic Reactions

- **Sneezing**: Frequent sneezing, particularly in moldy environments

- **Itchy Eyes**: Red, itchy, or watery eyes

- **Skin Rashes**: Hives or rashes on the skin

- **Postnasal Drip**: Mucus accumulation in the back of the throat

Asthma Symptoms

- **Asthma Attacks**: Increased frequency and severity of asthma attacks

- **Chest Tightness**: A feeling of tightness or pressure in the chest

- **Worsening Asthma**: Aggravation of existing asthma symptoms

Chronic Fatigue

- **Persistent Fatigue**: Constant tiredness or lethargy

- **Weakness**: General weakness and lack of energy

Headaches and Sinus Issues

- **Frequent Headaches**: Regular or persistent headaches that can vary in intensity

- **Sinus Congestion**: Blocked or stuffy sinuses

- **Sinusitis**: Inflammation or infection of the sinuses

Eye Irritation

- **Red Eyes**: Redness and inflammation in the eyes

- **Watery Eyes**: Excessive tearing or watery eyes

- **Itchy Eyes**: Persistent itching around the eyes

Cognitive and Neurological Symptoms

- **Memory Issues**: Difficulty remembering things or brain fog

- **Concentration Problems**: Trouble focusing or concentrating on tasks

- **Mood Changes**: Irritability, anxiety, or depression

Skin Symptoms

- **Rashes**: Red, itchy, or inflamed skin

- **Hives**: Raised, itchy welts on the skin

- **Skin Infections**: Infections of external auditory canal, nasal cavities, and cornea

Digestive Issues

- **Nausea**: Feeling nauseous or sick to the stomach

- **Vomiting**: Episodes of vomiting

- **Diarrhea**: Frequent loose or watery stools

Immune System Effects

- **Increased Infections**: More frequent respiratory infections or illnesses

- **Weakened Immune Response**: General reduction in immune system efficiency

Risk Factors and Sensitivity

Certain groups are more sensitive to mold exposure, including:

- **Individuals with Asthma**: People with preexisting respiratory conditions are more prone to severe symptoms

- **Allergy Sufferers**: Those with mold allergies experience heightened allergic reactions

- **Immunocompromised Individuals**: People with weakened immune systems are at higher risk for severe health effects

- **Infants and Children**: Young children are more susceptible to respiratory issues from mold exposure

- **Elderly**: Older adults may experience more severe health impacts due to a generally weaker immune system

- **Chronic Inflammation**: Overworked immune systems are more susceptible

- **Diet**: Mold can develop during food processing or storage, especially in items such as corn, cocoa, coffee, rice, grains, and nuts

Health Impacts On Pets

Respiratory Issues

- Pets, like humans, can develop respiratory problems from inhaling mold spores

- Symptoms include coughing, sneezing, and labored breathing

- Pets with pre-existing conditions are particularly vulnerable

Toxic Effects

- Pets are susceptible to the toxic effects of mycotoxins, which can cause vomiting, diarrhea, lethargy, and liver damage

- Ingesting contaminated food is a common way pets are exposed to mycotoxins

Neurological Effects

- Mycotoxins can affect the nervous system, leading to symptoms such as tremors, seizures, and changes in behavior or coordination

Myth:
You'd know if mold was making you sick it's obvious.

Fact:
Mold exposure symptoms like fatigue, sinus infections, or brain fog mimic allergies, a cold, or stress, often leading to misdiagnosis.

- Acute poisoning can be fatal if not treated promptly

Skin and Eye Irritation

- Pets may develop skin rashes and eye irritation from direct contact with mold or mold-contaminated surfaces

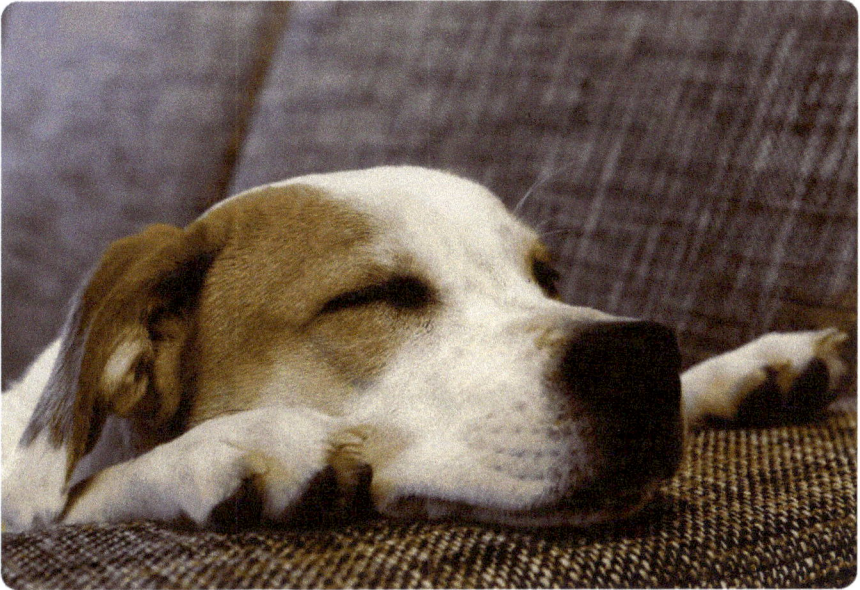

Why Misdiagnosis Happens & What to Do About it

Patients are often treated for colds during winter instead of mold-related illnesses, leading to prolonged exposure and worsening symptoms.

Mold-related illnesses can have symptoms that overlap with common colds or seasonal allergies:

- Respiratory Symptoms: Coughing, sneezing, nasal congestion, sore throat, or wheezing can look like a viral infection.

- Systemic Symptoms: Fatigue, headaches, brain fog, or muscle aches might be dismissed as part of a cold or flu.

- Seasonal Timing: Winter, when colds are rampant, also increases indoor mold growth due to humidity from heating, poor ventilation, or dampness—yet doctors may not think of mold first.

- Lack of Awareness: Many general practitioners aren't trained to recognize mold-related illnesses like Chronic Inflammatory Response Syndrome (CIRS) or fungal infections, especially if they're not common in their practice area.

Myth:
Mold testing is expensive and complicated.

Fact:
Simple DIY kits or visual checks can start the process; pros step in for tough cases.

Prolonged misdiagnosis can lead to ongoing exposure, worsening symptoms like asthma, sinus infections, or even neurological issues if mycotoxins (toxins produced by certain molds) are involved.

Steps to Prevent Misdiagnosis

Here's what you can do to advocate for yourself and ensure mold exposure is considered:

1. Document Your Symptoms and Environment

- Track Symptoms: Keep a detailed log of your symptoms, including when they started, their severity, and any patterns (e.g., worse at home, better when away). Note if symptoms persist beyond a typical cold (7-10 days) or don't respond to cold treatments like decongestants.

    - Mold-related symptoms might include: persistent sinus issues, shortness of breath, skin rashes, brain fog, joint pain, or sensitivity to light/smells.

- Assess Your Environment: Look for signs of mold in your home (e.g., musty smells, visible mold, water damage). Mention this to your doctor—exposure history is key. For example, "I've noticed black spots on my bathroom ceiling, and my symptoms started around the same time."

- Share Context: Tell your doctor if symptoms improve when you leave the suspected environment (e.g., on vacation) or worsen when you return. This can be a big clue for mold-related illness.

2. Be Proactive in Your Doctor's Visit

- Describe Symptoms Clearly: Avoid vague terms like "I feel sick." Instead, say, "I've had a cough and sinus pressure for 6 weeks, plus brain fog and fatigue, and cold medicine isn't helping." Highlight unusual symptoms (e.g., neurological issues, rashes) that don't fit a typical cold.

- Mention Mold Exposure: Directly bring up your concern about mold. For example, "I'm worried this might be related to mold in my home—can we test for that?" Doctors may not consider mold unless prompted.

- Ask About Misdiagnosis: Politely ask, "Could this be something other than a cold, like a reaction to mold? My symptoms aren't improving, and I've read that mold can cause similar issues." This shows you're informed and encourages the doctor to think beyond the obvious.

3. Insist on Specific Tests

If your doctor is leaning toward a cold diagnosis but you suspect mold, you can request tests to rule out or confirm mold-related illness. Here are some to discuss:

- **Allergy Testing:**

    - What It Does: Identifies if you're allergic to specific molds (e.g., Aspergillus, Penicillium). Skin prick tests or blood tests (like IgE testing) can show mold sensitivities.

    - Why It Helps: Positive results can link your symptoms to mold exposure, prompting further investigation.

    - What to Say: "Can we do an allergy test to see if I'm reacting to mold? I've been in a damp environment, and I think that might be the cause."

- **Mycotoxin Testing:**

    - What It Does: Tests for mycotoxins (toxins produced by molds like Stachybotrys or Aspergillus) in your body, usually via urine or blood. Labs like RealTime Laboratories offer mycotoxin panels.

- Why It Helps: Detects if toxic molds are affecting your health, which can cause systemic symptoms beyond a cold.

- What to Say: "I've read that mold can produce mycotoxins that make you sick—can we test for that in my urine or blood?"

- **Inflammatory Markers (for CIRS):**

  - What It Does: Tests for markers of Chronic Inflammatory Response Syndrome (CIRS), often linked to mold exposure. Key tests include:

    - C4a (complement protein, often elevated in mold illness).

    - TGF-beta 1 (transforming growth factor, linked to inflammation).

    - MMP-9 (matrix metalloproteinase, another inflammation marker).

  - Why It Helps: Elevated levels can indicate your body is reacting to biotoxins like mold, distinguishing it from a viral infection.

  - What to Say: "I've heard mold can cause Chronic Inflammatory Response Syndrome—can we test for markers like C4a or TGF-beta 1 to see if that's what's going on?"

- **Sinus Culture or Nasal Swab:**

  - What It Does: Checks for fungal infections in your sinuses (e.g., fungal sinusitis), which can mimic cold symptoms but persist longer.

- Why It Helps: Mold can colonize the sinuses, causing chronic issues that won't resolve with cold treatments.

- What to Say: "My sinus issues aren't going away—can we do a nasal swab to check for a fungal infection?"

- **Blood Work for Immune Response:**

  - What It Does: Tests for elevated IgG or IgM antibodies to molds, indicating exposure or infection. A complete blood count (CBC) can also show if your immune system is overactive (e.g., high eosinophils, common in allergic responses).

  - Why It Helps: Confirms if your body is reacting to mold rather than a virus.

  - What to Say: "Can we do blood work to check for mold antibodies or an immune response that might explain my symptoms?"

4. Seek a Specialist if Needed

- Who to See: If your primary doctor dismisses mold concerns or tests come back inconclusive but you're still symptomatic, consider seeing:

  - An allergist (for mold allergy testing).

  - An environmental medicine specialist (experts in mold-related illness).

  - A functional medicine doctor (often familiar with CIRS and mycotoxin issues).

- What to Say: "I'm still concerned about mold exposure—can you refer me to a specialist who deals with environmental illnesses?"

- Why It Helps: Specialists are more likely to recognize mold-related conditions and order advanced tests like those for CIRS or mycotoxins.

5. Test Your Environment

- Home Mold Testing: While waiting for medical tests, test your home for mold to strengthen your case. Use a DIY mold test kit (available online) or hire a professional to check for mold spores and humidity levels.

- Share Results: Bring test results to your doctor—e.g., "I had my home tested, and it showed high levels of Aspergillus. Could that be causing my symptoms?"

- Why It Helps: Concrete evidence of mold exposure can push your doctor to take your concerns seriously and guide their testing.

6. Address Mold Exposure Immediately

- Reduce Exposure: While pursuing a diagnosis, take steps to minimize mold exposure (e.g., clean visible mold with vinegar or hydrogen peroxide, use a dehumidifier, improve ventilation). This can help your symptoms and provide a clue—if symptoms improve after reducing exposure, it supports a mold-related diagnosis.

- Document Changes: Note if symptoms change after addressing mold, and share this with your doctor: "Since I cleaned the mold in my bathroom, my cough has improved—does that suggest it's mold-related?"

What to Insist On

When speaking with your doctor, be polite but firm. Here's a script to guide the conversation:

- "I'm concerned my symptoms might be related to mold exposure, not a cold, because they've lasted longer than expected and I've noticed mold in my home. Can we test for mold allergies, mycotoxins, or inflammatory markers like C4a to rule it out? I'd also like to check for a fungal infection in my sinuses, since my congestion won't go away."

If your doctor pushes back, you can add:

- "I understand colds are common, but my symptoms aren't improving with typical treatments, and I've read that mold can cause similar issues. I'd really like to explore this possibility to avoid prolonged exposure."

Additional Tips

- Bring Research: If your doctor isn't familiar with mold illness, bring a printout of reputable sources (e.g., CDC on mold health effects, or studies on CIRS) to show you've done your homework.

- Be Persistent: If initial tests are negative but you're still symptomatic, don't give up. Mold-related illnesses can be complex and may require multiple tests or a specialist's input.

- Monitor Symptoms: If new symptoms arise (e.g., neurological issues, severe fatigue), report them immediately—they could indicate a more serious mold-related condition.

> **Myth:**
> A little mold on a cutting board is no big deal—just wash it off.
>
> **Fact:**
> Mold can sink deep into porous wood, especially in knife grooves; light spots might be scrubbed out with vinegar, but extensive growth means it's time to toss it.

Mold Testing & Indoor Air Quality (IAQ): A Clear Guide

Mold States

Mold exists in three primary states:

- **Sporing** – Actively releasing spores into the air, which can be detected by air quality tests

- **Dormant** – Inactive but still present; can become active when conditions allow

- **Growing** – Actively spreading but not necessarily releasing spores, making it harder to detect with standard air tests

False Negatives

Because mold is not always sporing, many air quality tests result in false negatives, even in environments with significant mold contamination.

Mold Identification

You cannot accurately identify mold by simply looking at it. Testing is necessary to determine the type and potential toxicity of mold in your environment.

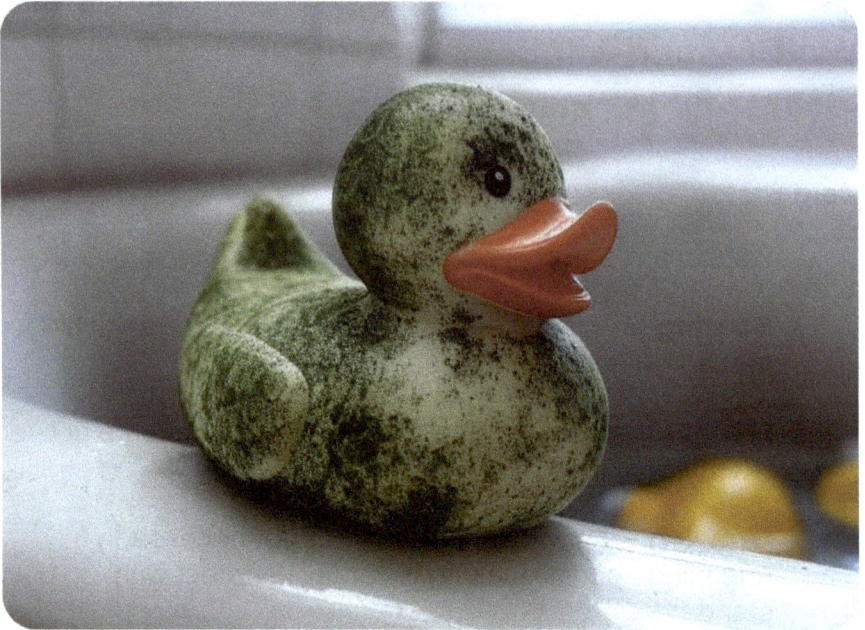

Mold-Related Statistics and Research

"The fungal kingdom includes as many as 6 million species and is remarkable in terms of the breadth and depth of its impact on global health, agriculture, biodiversity, ecology, manufacturing, and biomedical research. More than 600 fungal species are associated with humans, either as commensals and members of our microbiome or as pathogens that cause some of the most lethal infectious diseases." - *One Health: Fungal Pathogens of Humans, Animals, and Plants*

"Human fungal infections cause more than 1.5 million deaths every year."
- *The pathobiology of human fungal infections*

Mold Testing: Purpose and Process

Mold testing identifies and measures mold types and levels in environments. Professional inspectors conduct testing to determine if remediation is needed and guide removal efforts.

Mold often grows in hidden areas, making professional inspection necessary.

Types of Environmental Testing

Visual Inspection

- Initial walkthrough looking for visible mold and risk factors (water damage, humidity)

- Must be combined with other methods for complete assessment

Air Quality Testing

- Collects air samples using spore traps for lab analysis

- Identifies mold species and spore concentration

- Limitations: Only detects actively sporing mold; may miss non-sporing mold

Myth:
A moldy shower curtain is fine after a rinse—it's just bathroom grime.

Fact:
Surface mold might wash off with vinegar, but if it's embedded in fabric or the smell persists, it's a spore factory—toss it to keep your bathroom safe.

Surface/Swab Testing

- Collects samples from moldy surfaces for lab identification

- Confirms mold presence but doesn't measure quantity

Moisture Testing

- Uses moisture meters and thermal imaging to detect excess humidity and hidden leaks

Bulk Sampling

- Takes samples of contaminated materials for lab analysis

PCR-Based Tests

- ERMI (Environmental Relative Moldiness Index)

  - DNA-based testing of dust samples

  - Provides ranking score of mold contamination level

- HERTSMI-2

  - Modified version of ERMI focusing on five most toxic mold species

  - Assesses home safety for sensitive individuals

- PCR (Polymerase Chain Reaction)

  - Analyzes mold DNA to provide contamination history

  - Guidelines suggest a score of 10 or below is safe

EMMA Test (Environmental Mold and Mycotoxin Assessment)

- PCR-based test detecting both mold DNA and mycotoxins

- More sensitive than air tests; detects mold regardless of sporing

- Identifies specific mold species and harmful toxins

- Best for health-focused assessments, especially for those with sensitivities

Personal Testing

- Bio-resonance: Uses frequency to test for mold in the body

- Urine Test: Detects specific mycotoxins

- Gene Testing: Checks for HLA-DR gene linked to mold illness

Timeline

- Inspection: Typically 1-2 hours for most homes

- Lab results: Usually available within 48 hours

- Remediation: Can take days to weeks depending on severity

Professional Considerations

- In some states, inspection and remediation must be performed by separate companies to avoid conflicts of interest

- Severe infestations may warrant relocation rather than remediation

Trust Your Intuition

Even if tests come back negative, listen to your body. If you don't feel well and suspect mold exposure, trust your gut and take action—seek additional testing, monitor symptoms, and consider a professional mold assessment. For specific guidance on requesting further testing and discussing mold exposure with your doctor, see the section "Why Misdiagnosis Happens & What to Do About It."

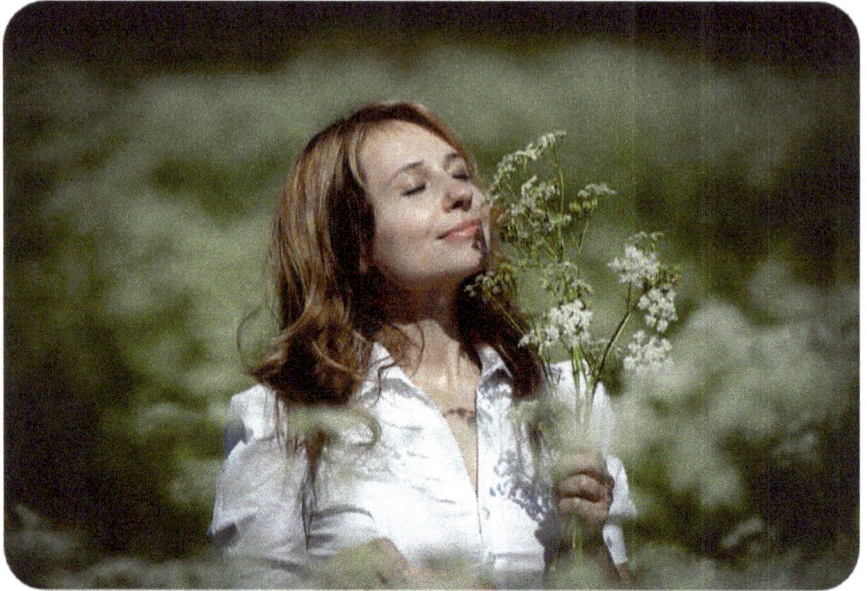

Where Mold Hides and How to Clean It

Mold can sneak into and thrive in many hidden corners of your home, growing unnoticed until it triggers health woes such as fatigue or coughs. Below, we'll spotlight common mold hideouts and show how hydrogen peroxide—a natural, powerful cleaner—can knock it out fast. While we use hydrogen peroxide as an example for its mold-killing punch, pick what works best for you—vinegar, borax, or store-bought options. Choose your weapon and fight back! When neutralizing and cleaning mold, **always** use protective clothing (mask, gloves, goggles, and clothes you can disinfect after or throw away) and ensure a well-ventilated area.

Myth:
A small mold spot on a mattress is harmless.

Fact:
Even a tiny spot can mean spores in the air you breathe; clean it with vinegar and dry it fast, but widespread mold or a musty smell means replacing it.

Common Household Hiding Spots

Water-Prone Areas

- **Behind Wallpaper:** Mold grows in the adhesive behind wallpaper, thriving in humid environments.
  Solution: Spray 3% hydrogen peroxide on affected areas, let sit for 10 minutes, wipe clean, and improve room ventilation.

- **Under Carpets and Pads:** Moisture trapped under carpets and pads fosters hidden mold growth.
  Solution: Lift carpet, spray 3% hydrogen peroxide on affected spots, dry thoroughly with fans, and address water sources.

- **Inside Walls**: Leaks or condensation inside walls create ideal mold conditions.
  Solution: Expose area (if possible), apply 3% hydrogen peroxide, let dry, and fix leaks to prevent recurrence.

- **Underneath Sinks:** Leaky pipes or condensation under sinks lead to mold in cabinets.
  Solution: Spray 3% hydrogen peroxide on moldy surfaces, wipe after 10 minutes, and repair leaks promptly.

- **On or Behind Drywall:** Drywall absorbs moisture, becoming a mold hotspot in basements or bathrooms.
  Solution: Mist 3% hydrogen peroxide on visible mold, wait 15 minutes, scrub lightly, and ventilate the area.

- **In Basements and Crawl Spaces:** Basements and crawl spaces, damp and poorly ventilated, are prime mold zones.
  Solution: Apply 3% hydrogen peroxide to surfaces, use a dehumidifier, and improve airflow with vents or fans.

- **Around Windows:** Condensation around windows causes mold on sills and frames.
  Solution: Spray 3% hydrogen peroxide, wipe after 10 minutes, and use weather stripping to reduce moisture.

- **In Chimneys:** Chimneys accumulate moisture and debris, promoting mold growth.
  Solution: Mist 3% hydrogen peroxide on accessible areas, clean debris, and ensure proper chimney venting.

- **In Attics:** Roof leaks or poor attic ventilation lead to mold on insulation or beams.
  Solution: Spray 3% hydrogen peroxide on moldy spots, dry with fans, and fix roof or add vents.

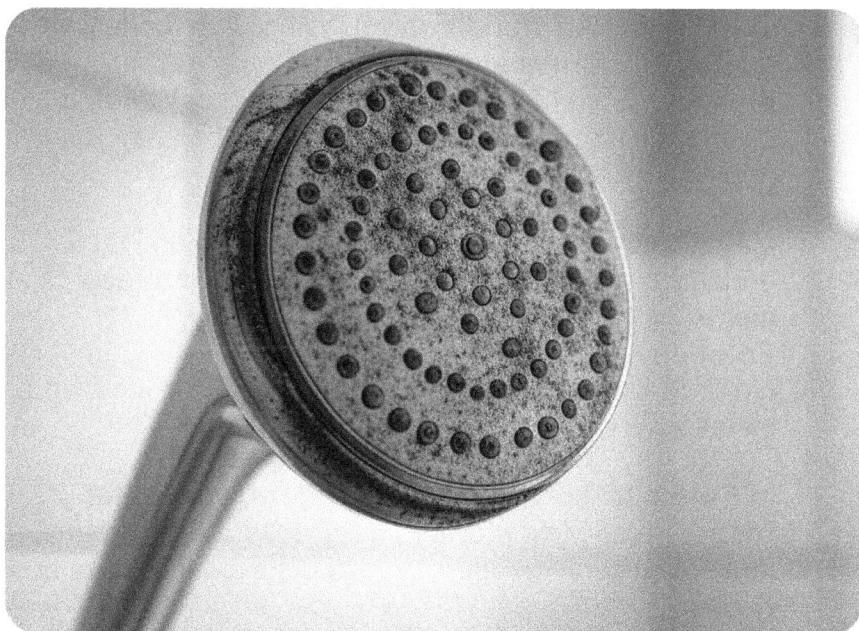

Appliances and Systems

- **In Air Conditioners and HVAC Systems:** Mold develops in air conditioners and HVAC systems, spreading spores through ducts.
  Solution: Clean coils and filters with 3% hydrogen peroxide, let sit for 10 minutes, rinse, and replace filters regularly.

- **In Washing Machines and Dishwashers:** Rubber seals and drawers in washing machines and dishwashers harbor mold from moisture.
  Solution: Wipe seals with 3% hydrogen peroxide, leave doors open to dry, and run an empty cycle with peroxide monthly.

- **In Refrigerator Drip Pans:** Refrigerator drip pans collect moisture and debris, fostering mold.
  Solution: Remove pan, soak with 3% hydrogen peroxide for 15 minutes, scrub, and dry completely.

- **On Window Air Conditioners:** Window air conditioners grow mold in filters and coils.
  Solution: Spray 3% hydrogen peroxide on filter and coils, wait 10 minutes, rinse, and air dry before reinstalling.

- **Under and Behind Appliances:** Moisture and food under or behind appliances like refrigerators breed mold.
  Solution: Pull appliances out, spray 3% hydrogen peroxide on floor and base, wipe after 10 minutes, and clean spills promptly.

- **In Coffee Makers, Juicers, Blenders, and Water Dispensers:** Mold grows in water reservoirs of coffee makers, juicers, blenders, and dispensers if not cleaned well.
  Solution: Fill the reservoir with 3% hydrogen peroxide, soak for 15 minutes, rinse thoroughly, and dry after each use.

- **In Ductwork:** Dust and moisture in ductwork lead to mold spread throughout the home.
  Solution: Use 3% hydrogen peroxide in a spray to clean accessible duct openings, and hire pros for full duct cleaning.

- **In Humidifiers:** Standing water in humidifiers becomes a mold breeding ground.
  Solution: Empty, soak tank with 3% hydrogen peroxide for 15 minutes, rinse, and clean weekly.

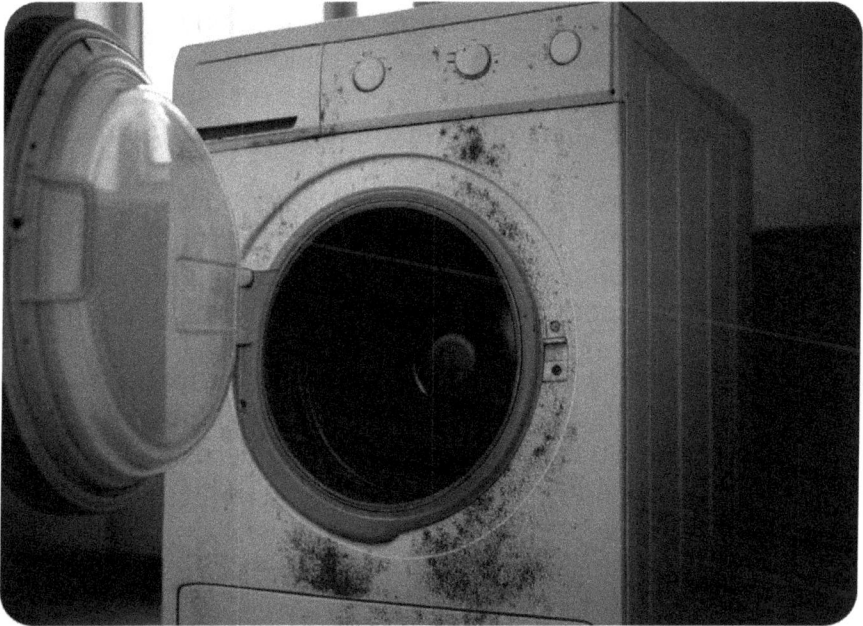

Everyday Items

- **In Hot Tubs and Water Features:** Stagnant or warm water in hot tubs and water features fosters mold on surfaces or in water.
  Solution: Add 3% hydrogen peroxide to water (1 cup per 100 gallons), scrub surfaces, and circulate to kill mold.

- **In Pools:** Warm, still water in pools—especially if neglected—breeds mold on tiles, liners, or in the water itself.
  Solution: Add 3% hydrogen peroxide (2 cups per 200 gallons), scrub tiles and edges with a brush, and run the filter 24 hours to kill mold.

- **On Houseplants:** Overwatering houseplants causes mold on soil or the plant itself.
  Solution: Spray soil with 1 tbsp 3% hydrogen peroxide per cup of water, reduce watering, and improve airflow.

- **Behind Furniture:** Furniture against poorly insulated walls traps moisture, leading to mold.
  Solution: Move furniture 2-3 inches out, spray wall with 3% hydrogen peroxide, wipe after 10 minutes, and dry.

- **In Pet Areas:** Moisture from pet water bowls or accidents creates mold on floors or bedding.
  Solution: Clean bowls with 3% hydrogen peroxide, spot-treat floors, dry thoroughly, and refresh bedding.

- **In Children's Plastic Bath Toys:** Water trapped in children's plastic bath toys leads to mold growth.
  Solution: Soak toys in 3% hydrogen peroxide for 15 minutes, rinse, dry, and seal openings with glue.

- **In Shower Curtains:** Shower curtains harbor mold from constant moisture exposure.
  Solution: Spray 3% hydrogen peroxide, let sit for 10 minutes, scrub, and hang to dry fully after showers.

- **In Books and Papers:** Books and papers stored in damp conditions become moldy.
  Solution: *Paper is delicate—hydrogen peroxide's moisture could damage pages or ink, while UV-C sanitizes surfaces without wetting. Direct exposure kills mold spores effectively on exposed areas.Use a UV-C wand or lamp (254 nm, ozone-free) over pages for 30-60 seconds per side in a well-ventilated area, then store with desiccant (a substance that promotes drying such as calcium oxide or silica gel). Avoid prolonged exposure to prevent yellowing.

- **On Ceiling Tiles:** Ceiling tiles in damp areas develop mold.
  Solution: Spray 3% hydrogen peroxide, wait 10 minutes, wipe, and replace if damage persists.

- **In Garage and Outdoor Equipment:** Garage and outdoor equipment in damp sheds grow mold.

Solution: Wipe tools with 3% hydrogen peroxide, dry thoroughly, and store with silica gel packs.

- **On Toothbrush Holders:** Residual water in toothbrush holders leads to mold.
  Solution: Soak holder in 3% hydrogen peroxide for 15 minutes, rinse, and dry after each use.

- **In Mattresses and Upholstery:** Sweat and spills on mattresses and upholstery foster mold.
  Solution: Spot-treat with 3% hydrogen peroxide, blot dry, and use a mattress protector.

- **In Potted Plant Saucers:** Water in potted plant saucers becomes a mold breeding ground.
  Solution: Empty saucer, wipe with 3% hydrogen peroxide, and avoid overwatering.

- **On Window Sills and Frames:** Condensation and leaks on window sills and frames cause mold.
  Solution: Spray 3% hydrogen peroxide, wipe after 10 minutes, and seal frames to stop leaks.

- **In Clogged Gutters:** Standing water in clogged gutters leads to mold on roofs and walls.
  Solution: Clear gutters, spray 3% hydrogen peroxide on moldy areas, and rinse with a hose.

- **In Carpets in Damp Areas:** Carpets in damp basements or bathrooms absorb moisture and grow mold.
  Solution: Spray 3% hydrogen peroxide, dry with fans, and consider removing if mold persists.

- **On Grout in Tiled Areas:** Grout in tiled areas harbors mold from constant moisture.
  Solution: Apply 3% hydrogen peroxide, scrub after 10 minutes, and reseal grout yearly.

- **On Pillows and Mattresses:** Moisture from sweat or spills on pillows and mattresses causes mold.
  Solution: Spot-treat with 3% hydrogen peroxide, air dry, and use breathable covers.

- **On Faucets and Shower Heads:** Frequent moisture on faucets and showerheads leads to mold.
  Solution: Wipe with 3% hydrogen peroxide, rinse after 10 minutes, and dry after use.

- **In Drains:** Drains' damp environment is perfect for mold colonization.
  Solution: Pour 3% hydrogen peroxide down the drain, let sit for 15 minutes, and flush with hot water.

- **On Shoes:** Wet shoes in dark closets develop mold.
  Solution: *The preference is to keep items made of porous material such as shoes dry. UV-C sanitizes surfaces without wetting. Direct exposure kills mold spores effectively on exposed areas. Use a UV-C wand or lamp (254 nm, ozone-free) inside and on shoes for 30-60 seconds in a well-ventilated area, then store with desiccant (a substance that promotes drying such as calcium oxide or silica gel).

- **On Furniture:** Furniture in humid conditions or against cold walls grows mold.

- **Solution:** Spray 3% hydrogen peroxide on non-porous parts, wipe after 10 minutes, and reposition for airflow. *For furniture made of porous materials such as fabric, use a UV-C wand or lamp (254 nm, ozone-free).

> **Tip:**
> Seal kid's bath toys—stop mold inside!

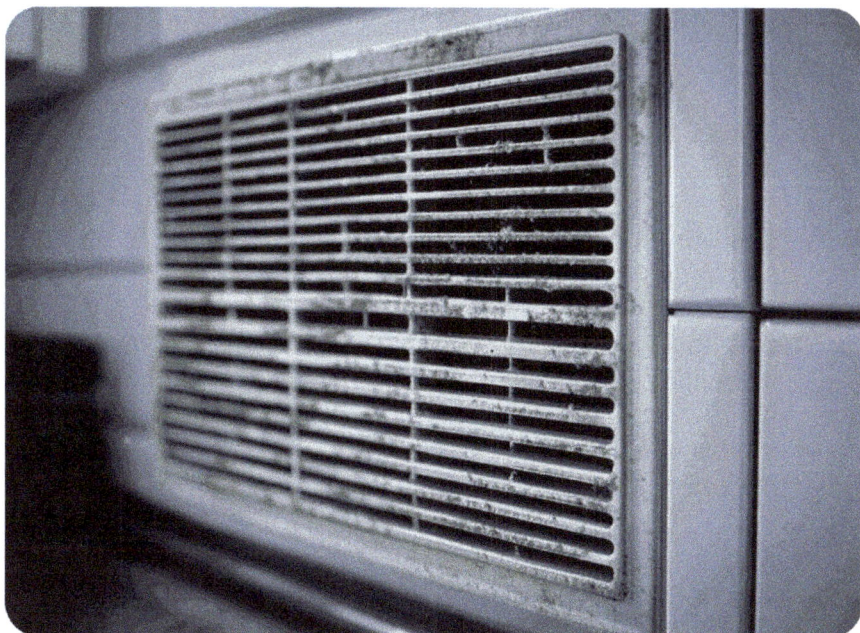

Environmental Factors

- **EMF Radiation**: Studies have shown electromagnetic field radiation may increase the growth rate of toxic mold.
  Consider:

  - Turning off WiFi and other electromagnetic devices when not in use, especially before sleep

  - Spending more time outside barefoot to ground yourself

  - Using EMF protection devices in high-radiation areas

Signs Of Mold Presence

Regular inspection for these signs can help you identify mold problems early:

- **Musty odors**: A persistent earthy, musty smell often indicates hidden mold

- **Water stains**: Discolored patches on walls, ceilings, or floors

- **Visible discoloration**: Black, green, or white spots on surfaces

- **Peeling wallpaper**: Wallpaper that's peeling or bubbling, especially at seams

- **Warped or cracked walls**: Structural changes indicating moisture damage

- **Increased allergy symptoms**: Worsening allergies when in specific areas of your home

- **Increasing fatigue or brain fog**: Cognitive symptoms that improve when away from home

- **Condensation**: Excessive moisture on windows, pipes, or walls

- **Bubbling paint**: Paint that bubbles or cracks due to moisture underneath

Tip:
Ventilate bathrooms daily—stale air breeds mold fast!

Preventing Mold Growth

Controlling mold is crucial for health, especially for vulnerable populations such as those with immune system disorders, hypersensitive individuals, pregnant women, newborns, the elderly, and cancer patients. When neutralizing and cleaning mold, **always** use protective clothing (mask, gloves, goggles, and clothes you can disinfect after or throw away) and ensure a well-ventilated area.

For Homes

- **Moisture Control**:

    - Keep indoor humidity below 50% using dehumidifiers if necessary

    - Fix leaks promptly (pipes, roofs, windows)

    - Dry wet areas within 24-48 hours

    - Use exhaust fans in kitchens and bathrooms

- **Ventilation Strategies**:

    - Regularly ventilate rooms, especially those with gas-fired appliances

    - Open windows in bathrooms and kitchens to reduce moisture

    - Create cross breezes to sweep stagnant air out daily

    - Ensure proper attic and crawl space ventilation

- **Laundry Practices**:

    - Avoid indoor drying: Dry clothes outside in fresh air and sunlight when possible

    - Towel care: Hang towels in a well-ventilated area after showering

    - Clean washing machine regularly, especially rubber seals

- **Cleaning Routines**:

    - Regular refrigerator maintenance: Wash refrigerator shelves and interior surfaces

    - Regular cleaning of bathrooms, kitchens, and basements with mold-inhibiting products

    - Vacuum carpets regularly using HEPA filters

    - Clean air ducts professionally if needed

- **Strategic Prevention**:

    - Use mold-resistant products when building or renovating (mold-resistant drywall, paint with mold inhibitors)

    - Improve air flow in problem areas

    - Reduce clutter, which can hold moisture and prevent airflow

    - Consider using air purifiers with HEPA filters

For Pets

- **Safe Food Storage**: Store pet food in dry, airtight containers and discard any moldy food

- **Regular Grooming**: Keep pets clean and dry, especially if they have been in damp environments

- **Clean Living Spaces**: Regularly clean and disinfect pet bedding, toys, and living areas

- **Moisture Control**: Clean up water spills from pet bowls promptly

- **Air Quality**: Ensure pet areas have adequate ventilation and air circulation

By being aware of these hidden and unexpected places, you can take steps to inspect, clean, and prevent mold growth, ensuring a healthier living environment for both you and your pets. Regular maintenance, proper ventilation, and controlling moisture are key to preventing mold from taking hold in these overlooked areas.

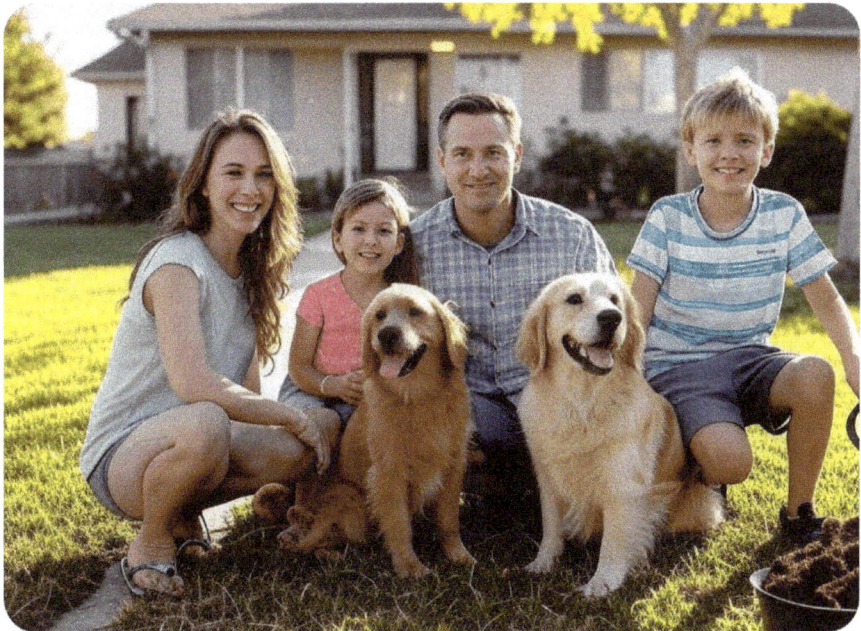

Suspect Mold? Your Action Plan

Dealing with mold requires a proactive, multi-faceted approach—stopping exposure, supporting your health, and preventing recurrence. This action plan provides immediate steps and a comprehensive recovery protocol, drawing from environmental science and holistic health strategies. Act swiftly, but don't panic; knowledge and consistency are your best tools.

Immediate Steps

When you suspect mold, time is critical. These initial actions help you assess the situation, protect yourself, and gather evidence for recovery or remediation.

1. **Document Everything**

    a. **Take Photos:** Capture clear, time-stamped images of visible mold, water damage, or damp areas. Photograph multiple angles and include context (e.g., affected rooms, furniture). These records are invaluable for insurance claims, remediation planning, or legal purposes.

    b. **Keep a Symptom Diary:** Log physical or mental symptoms (e.g., fatigue, respiratory issues, brain fog) with dates, times, and severity. Note patterns—like worsening symptoms indoors versus outdoors—to link health effects to your environment.

    c. **Record Dates of Water Damage:** Pinpoint when leaks, floods, or humidity spikes occurred. Even small incidents (e.g., a spill left unattended) can trigger mold growth within 24–48 hours, per EPA research. This timeline helps identify the source and scope.

2. Test Your Environment

a. **ERMI Test:** The Environmental Relative Moldiness Index (ERMI) uses DNA-based analysis of dust to identify 36 mold species, offering a historical snapshot of mold levels. Collect samples with a vacuum attachment or Swiffer cloth from high-traffic areas (e.g., living room, bedroom). Costs range from $290–$350 via labs like Mycometrics or EnviroBiomics. Compare results to the national database (scores above 5 suggest elevated moldiness), but note the EPA considers ERMI a research tool, not a definitive diagnostic. Pair it with other tests for clarity.

b. **Air Quality Testing:** Spore trap air sampling measures current airborne mold levels. Hire a professional to take indoor and outdoor samples (e.g., using Air-O-Cell cassettes) for comparison. Normal indoor levels should not exceed outdoor baselines significantly. Results are quicker than ERMI but less comprehensive historically.

c. **Surface Sampling:** Swabs or tape lifts from visible mold or suspect surfaces pinpoint specific species. This is ideal for confirming toxicity (e.g., Stachybotrys, "black mold") and guiding remediation. Labs like EMSL Analytical offer affordable kits ($50–$100). Combine with ERMI for a fuller picture.

3. Protect Yourself

a. **Use Air Purifiers:** Deploy HEPA-filter air purifiers (minimum MERV 13 rating) in affected areas to trap mold spores. Models like the Alen BreatheSmart ($400–$700) are effective for larger spaces. Run continuously during cleanup.

b. **Wear N95 Masks During Cleaning:** N95 respirators block 95% of airborne particles, including mold spores. Fit-test the mask for a tight seal—cloth masks won't suffice. Wear gloves and goggles too; mold can irritate skin and eyes.

c. **Consider Temporary Relocation if Severe:** If mold levels are high (e.g., ERMI >10, visible growth extensive), or symptoms are debilitating, relocate temporarily. Sensitive individuals (e.g., with asthma, CIRS) may react to even low exposure.

d. **Take a Bio-Resonance Health Scan:** This alternative method can detect mold-related stress in your body via electromagnetic frequencies. ($200–$500). Use as a supplementary tool, not a primary diagnostic. Additionally, consult with a mold-literate health specialist to create a tailored health plan for your unique needs.

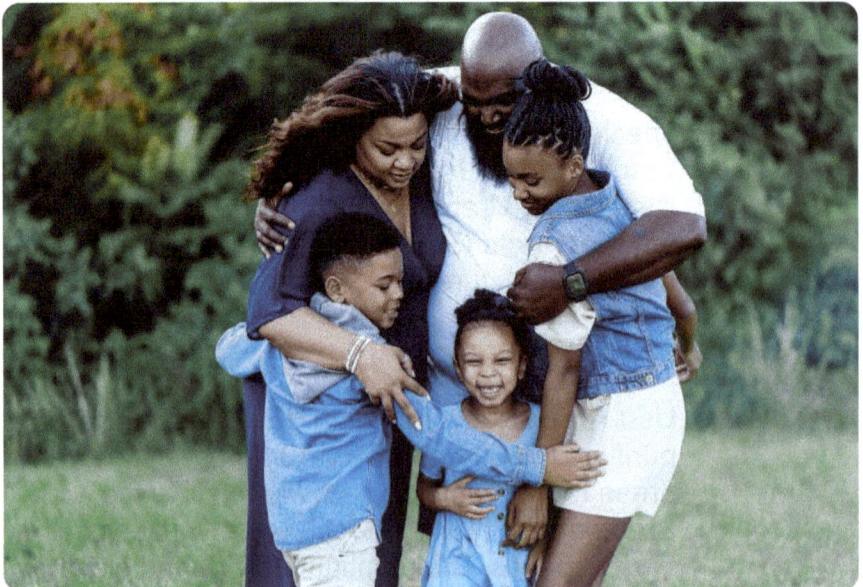

The Recovery Protocol

Recovering from mold exposure involves three interconnected steps: stopping the source, supporting your body, and cleaning your environment. Each builds on the previous, creating a solid path to lasting health. When neutralizing and cleaning mold, **always** use protective clothing (mask, gloves, goggles, and clothes you can disinfect after or throw away) and ensure a well-ventilated area.

Step 1: Stop the Exposure

Mold needs moisture, stagnant air, and organic material to grow. Eliminate these to halt its spread.

- **Fix Water Leaks**: Check plumbing, roofs, and appliances with a moisture meter ($20–$50); readings above 15% signal risk. Repair leaks within 24–48 hours—EPA research shows mold can start growing this fast on wet surfaces.

- **Remove Contaminated Materials**: Discard porous items (e.g., drywall, carpet) with visible mold or prolonged water exposure, sealing them in plastic bags to trap spores. Clean non-porous surfaces (e.g., tile, glass) instead.

- **Dry Damp Areas**: Use dehumidifiers (target 30–50% humidity) and fans to dry wet spots within 24–48 hours. Desiccants like silica gel work in small spaces.

- **Improve Ventilation**: Install exhaust fans (50+ CFM) in bathrooms and kitchens. Ventilate daily for 15–30 minutes with open windows when outdoor humidity is below 50%, monitored by a hygrometer ($10–$20).

- **Hang Up Wet Items**: Dry towels and clothes on racks or lines immediately—mold thrives on damp fabric.

- **Use Sunlight**: Open blinds daily for 1+ hour; UV rays naturally inhibit mold, per CDC guidance. Balance with ventilation in humid seasons.

- **Reduce EMF**: Some evidence suggests that disharmonic electromagnetic fields (EMF) stress immunity and can promote microbial growth in damp settings. As a precaution, turn off Wi-Fi at night and limit device use near water-damaged areas. If you cannot switch off the Wi-Fi, wrap your phones and electronics with a copper mesh to dampen the signal when not used.

> **Tip:**
> Wash pet beds weekly—damp fur breeds hidden mold!

Step 2: Support Your Body With Personalized Care for Mold-Related Health

Mold, particularly mycotoxin-producing varieties, can place significant stress on your body's systems. Supporting detoxification and resilience through diet, supplements, and therapies help. The options listed below are general suggestions for readers to explore further.

While the following approaches are helpful for many, consulting a mold-literate health practitioner is essential to create a tailored plan suited to your unique needs and circumstances.

- **Diet Adjustments**

    - **Cut Sugar From Your Diet:** Reduces inflammation and starves yeast/mold in your gut. Skip sweets, sodas, and refined carbohydrates.

    - **Avoid Processed Foods:** Preservatives burden the liver, key for mycotoxin clearance. Choose whole foods.

    - **Boost Vegetables:** Leafy greens and cruciferous veggies (e.g., kale, broccoli, brussel sprouts) support liver detox; antioxidants (e.g., berries) fight oxidative stress.

- **Hydrate:** Drink 6–10 cups of filtered water daily to flush toxins.

- **Lemon water:** Drink freshly squeezed lemon or lime room temperature water with zest first thing upon waking to support your liver and alkalize your system. (**Do not** start your day with caffeine, sugar, fats, or proteins.)

- **Celery juicing:** Drink fresh celery juice every morning (30-60 minutes after having lemon water) and in the evening to support the rejuvenation of your cells.

- **Eat Mindfully:** Slow down, enjoy your food, feel appreciation for it. Don't use anything digital while eating. Stop eating once you are 80% full, chew 20–30 times per bite (minimum), and avoid liquids during meals to aid digestion (wait 1 hour to drink a beverage before/after eating).

- **Supplements**

  - **Kidney and Liver Detoxification:** Support your kidneys with bioflavonoids first and a few hours later take a binder to aid your liver in detoxing. Consult a health specialist to ensure your liver and kidneys are getting additional support as per your unique needs and situation.

  - **Binders and Their Role in Mycotoxin Elimination**—Binders, including insoluble fibers such as flax seeds, psyllium husks, or activated charcoal assist in the removal of mycotoxins by capturing bile in the intestines. After mycotoxins are absorbed through respiratory passages or skin and processed by the liver into bile, these binders facilitate the excretion of bile-bound toxins, preventing their reabsorption into the body. Incorporating 2-4 tablespoons daily with meals supports this process efficiently, leveraging the natural release of bile during digestion. Ingest several hours after taking bioflavonoids.

*For a detailed analysis of each binder, see the section "Binders for Mycotoxin Elimination: Evaluation and Ranking."

○ **Antifungals for Nasal Mold Relief**—Using an antifungal such as grapefruit seed extract or colloidal silver in a nasal spray may help reduce mold growth lining your nasal passages, a common entry point for spores in moldy environments. By targeting this area, it can support respiratory health and limit mycotoxin exposure.

○ **Magnesium for Detox Support**— Taking a magnesium supplement, such as magnesium glycinate or citrate, can support your body while detoxing from mold exposure. Mold-related illnesses often cause inflammation, fatigue, and stress on the nervous system due to mycotoxin buildup. Magnesium helps by supporting cellular detoxification, reducing inflammation, and calming the nervous system, which can ease symptoms like muscle aches, brain fog, and anxiety. Aim for 200-400 mg daily (consult your health practitioner for the right dose), and pair it with a nutrient-rich diet to aid your body's recovery.

○ **Homeopathics for Mold Symptom Support**—Homeopathic remedies, tailored by a trained practitioner, may help alleviate symptoms of mold exposure by stimulating your body's natural healing response. These gentle treatments could target issues like respiratory discomfort or fatigue.

- Vitamin C (Buffered or Liposomal) for Immune Support—Supplementing with buffered or liposomal vitamin C can enhance immune resilience against mold-related stress, thanks to its antioxidant power and improved absorption. Buffered forms are gentler on the stomach, while liposomal delivery boosts bioavailability

- **Therapies**

  - Infrared Sauna for Detoxification—Infrared saunas promote sweating, which may help your body expel mycotoxins through the skin, reducing the toxic load from mold exposure. Sessions of 20–30 minutes, 2–3 times weekly, can support this process (cost: $50–$100 per session or $1,000+ for a home unit); consult a practitioner to ensure it aligns with your health goals.

  - Hyperbaric Oxygen Therapy (HBOT) for Recovery—HBOT boosts oxygen levels in your tissues, potentially accelerating healing and reducing inflammation caused by mold-related damage. Typically involving 1–2 hour sessions ($100–$200 each), it may enhance cellular repair—consult a specialist to determine if it's suitable for your condition.

  - Bio-Resonance: Uses gentle frequencies to assist the body in detoxing. ($200–$500/session). Use as a supplementary tool in combination with other detox and recovery strategies.

- **Boost Well-Being**

  - Detoxing from mold can be stressful, and stress weakens your immunity, slowing recovery. Lift your spirits to support healing. Smile, hug loved ones, and laugh often—these simple acts release feel-good hormones like oxytocin and serotonin, boosting your mood and resilience. Daily exercise, such as a 30-minute walk in nature, to promote detoxing, strengthens your immune system, and helps you thrive. Spend time at the beach, breathing in salty air, which can clear your respiratory passages and calm your mind with the sound of waves. Other soul-nourishing practices include watching a sunrise or sunset, gardening to connect with the earth, or listening to uplifting music—whatever feeds your spirit and brings you joy.

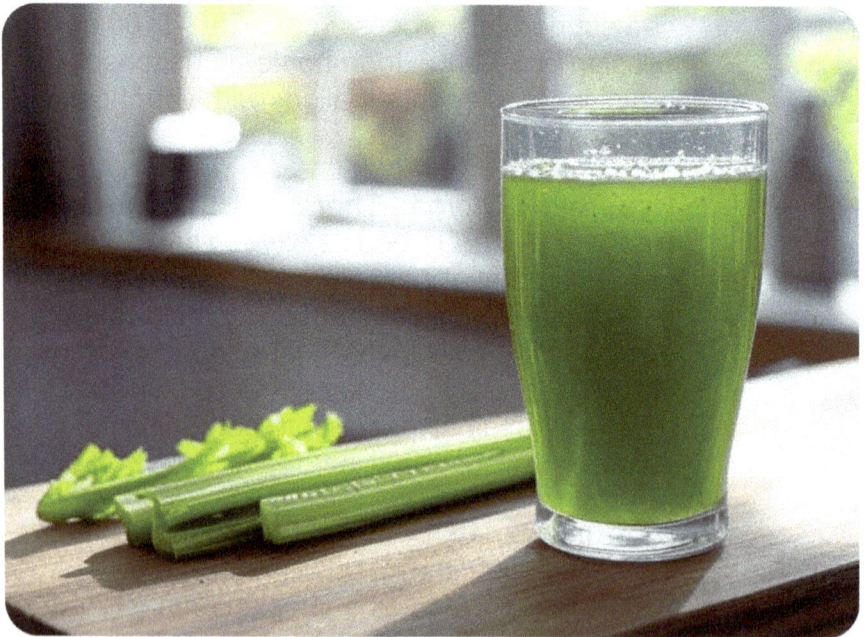

Binders for Mycotoxin Elimination: Evaluation and Ranking

Binders help remove mycotoxins by capturing bile in the intestines, where toxins are processed after being absorbed through respiratory passages or skin and filtered by the liver. Incorporating binders into your daily routine can prevent reabsorption of these toxins, supporting your body's detox process during mold recovery. Below, we evaluate and rank four binders based on their effectiveness and inflammatory impact, providing practical guidance for use. Always consult a mold-literate health practitioner to tailor your protocol, and take binders several hours after bioflavonoids to avoid interference.

1. Activated Charcoal

- **Effectiveness:** Very High—Top binder, adsorbs a wide range of mycotoxins (e.g., aflatoxins, ochratoxin), per studies (e.g., Food Additives & Contaminants, 2007). Used in detox protocols (e.g., Dr. Neil Nathan's Toxic).

- **Inflammation:** Very Low—Non-digestible, passes through without fermentation or irritation. Can bind nutrients if overused, so time away from meals (1-2 hours).

- **Dose:** 500 mg to 1 g daily—capsules or powder ($10-$15).

- **Pros:** Potent, mold-specific, gentle on the gut.

- **Cons:** Not food-based—less nutritive than flax.

- **Why It Ranks Highest:** Highest binding capacity, grabbing most mycotoxins with zero inflammation risk. Best for acute mold detox.

- **Use:** Take 500 mg 1-2 hours before meals—pairs well with flax for added nutrition.

2. Bentonite Clay

- **Effectiveness:** Very High—Strong adsorbent, binds mycotoxins (e.g., aflatoxins), per research (e.g., Applied Clay Science, 2015). Common in mold recovery protocols.

- **Inflammation:** Low—Soothes gut lining, non-fermentable. Must mix with water—gritty if not hydrated.

- **Dose:** 1 tsp in 8 oz water daily ($10-$15/bag).

- **Pros:** Powerful, gut-healing, affordable.

- **Cons:** Messier than flax—needs prep.

- **Why It Ranks High:** Matches charcoal's binding power, adds gut-soothing minerals, and has low inflammation risk—ideal for sensitive systems.

- **Use:** Mix 1 tsp in 8 oz water, once daily—stir well.

3. Flax Seeds

- **Effectiveness:** Moderate to High—Rich in soluble fiber (mucilage) and insoluble fiber, binds mycotoxins moderately well, per holistic sources (e.g., Dr. Jill Crista's Break the Mold). Studies show flax's lignans and fiber trap toxins like heavy metals and some mycotoxins (e.g., aflatoxins).

- **Inflammation:** Low—Generally anti-inflammatory due to omega-3s (ALA), supports gut healing. Easy to digest when ground, though whole seeds may irritate sensitive guts.

- **Dose:** 2 tbsp daily (~5-6g fiber), gentle and effective ($5/bag).

- **Pros:** Affordable, nutrient-rich, versatile.

- **Cons:** Limited binding strength compared to specialized binders like charcoal.

- **Why It Ranks Well:** Solid binding capacity, anti-inflammatory omega-3s, and easy digestion when ground make it a go-to—versatile and gentle for most.

- **Use:** Sprinkle 2 tbsp daily on food—great for adding nutrition alongside stronger binders.

4. Psyllium Husks

- **Effectiveness:** Moderate to High—Soluble fiber forms a gel, traps mycotoxins (e.g., ochratoxin A) well, per gut health research (e.g., Nutrients, 2019). Broad binding potential.

- **Inflammation:** Low to Moderate—Gentle for most, softens stool, reduces irritation. High fiber (5g/tsp) can cause bloating if not hydrated well, especially in sensitive guts.

- **Dose:** 1-2 tsp in water—needs lots of liquid ($10/bag).

- **Pros:** Cheap, widely available, stool-regulating.

- **Cons:** Requires careful hydration—less convenient than flax.

- **Why It Ranks Mid-Tier:** Good binding and generally gentle, but a slight bloating risk drops it below flax for mold-sensitive individuals.

- **Use:** Mix 1 tsp in water, drink quickly, and follow with more water.

Step 3: Clean Your Environment

Spot mold, stop it fast, and clean smart—effective cleaning neutralizes mold without spreading spores. Match your approach to the problem's size and severity, using tools from this guide. Remember to wear protective clothing (gloves, mask, goggles, old clothing you can disinfect or throw away).

For Severe Mold

- **The Issue:** Mold over 10 sq ft (EPA guideline), inside walls, in HVAC systems, or causing intense symptoms (e.g., breathing issues, fatigue).

- **Solution:** Hire certified pros (e.g., IICRC or ACAC remediators)—DIY risks spreading spores or worsening health. For extreme cases (e.g., structural mold), relocate temporarily; it's safer than fighting an invisible enemy.

- **Possessions Tip:** Take only essentials when leaving. Spores hitch rides on clothes and furniture—wash what you keep with Borax or discard to avoid cross-contamination.

For Minor Mold

- **The Issue:** Small patches (under 10 sq ft) on surfaces like tile, grout, or toys.

- **Solution:** Neutralize mold first—soap and water alone scatter spores. Here's how:
  - **UV-C Lights**: Use ozone-free 254 nm lamps (e.g., Medify MA-40 UV-C, $100-$150) to kill mold DNA on dry surfaces like books or toothbrush holders. Run 15-30 seconds per area, avoiding skin/eye exposure—check safety instructions.

  - **Hydrogen Peroxide:** Spray 3% food-grade solution ($2-$6/quart), wait 10 minutes, scrub, and wipe dry. Kills up to 90% of mold species—wear gloves, mask, goggles, and ventilate to avoid irritation.

- o **Vinegar:** Spray 5-8% distilled white vinegar ($2-$5/gallon), wait 1 hour, scrub, and rinse. Kills 82% of molds—use gloves and ventilate for the smell; 20% vinegar boosts power for stubborn spots.

- **Clean Safely:** After neutralizing, scrub with soap and water, then use a HEPA vacuum (e.g., Shop-Vac, $100-$200) to trap spores. Empty outside into sealed bags to keep mold out of your air.

Bonus Tools

- **Colloidal Silver:** Add 5-10 drops to humidifier water ($10-$30/bottle) for antimicrobial support—keeps mold from spreading through mist.

- **Bio-Resonance:** Do some sessions ($200-$500) to aid detox if mold lingers in your body—gentle frequencies can assist the body in detoxing.

Prevention Strategies

Prevention is cheaper and easier than recovery. Build these habits into your routine and maintain your home seasonally.

Daily Habits

- **Run Bathroom Fans:** Exhaust moisture during and 20 minutes after showers (50–100 CFM fans, $30–$100).

- **Use Dehumidifiers:** Keep humidity below 50% in basements, bathrooms, and kitchens ($150–$300/unit). Empty tanks daily.

- **Check for Leaks:** Inspect under sinks, around windows, and near appliances weekly. Fix drips immediately.

- **Clean Air Filters:** Replace HVAC filters (MERV 8–13) every 1–3 months ($10–$20 each) to trap spores and maintain airflow.

- **Maintain Ventilation**: Crack windows or run fans daily to cycle fresh air. Stagnation breeds mold.

- **Hang Up Towels and Clothes:** Dry wet items within hours—don't let them sit damp.

- **Let in Sunlight:** Open blinds daily; UV light deters mold naturally.

- **Air Out Your Home:** Ventilate 15–30 minutes daily, even in cold months, to refresh air.

- **Boost Well-Being:** Smile, hug loved ones, and laugh—stress weakens immunity. Exercise daily (e.g., 30-minute walks) to support detox, a strong immune system, and thriving.

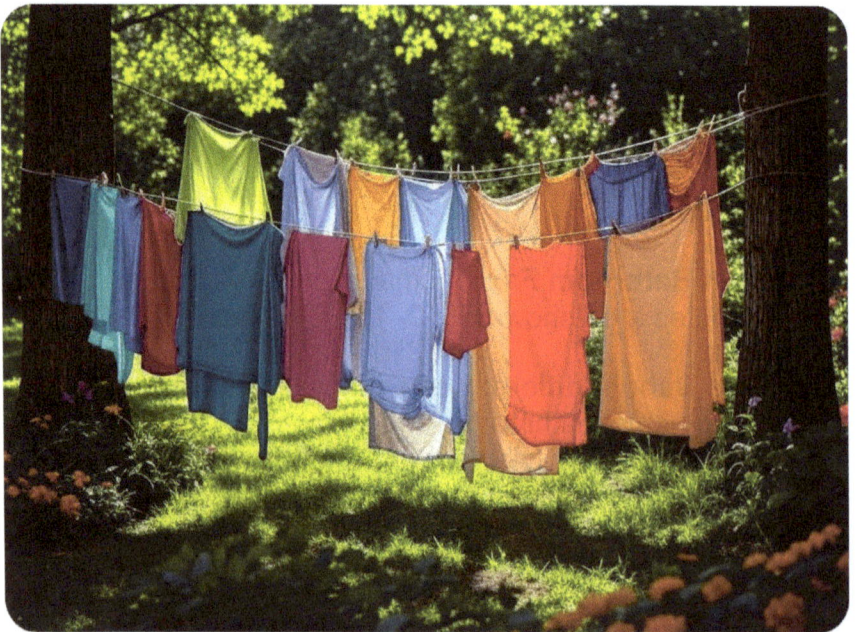

Seasonal Maintenance

- **Check Roof and Gutters:** Clear debris and repair leaks in spring/fall to prevent water intrusion ($100–$500 if professional).

- **Inspect Window Seals:** Re-caulk cracks annually ($10–$20) to block moisture entry.

- **Clean Air Ducts:** Hire pros every 3–5 years ($300–$500) to remove dust and spores. DIY vent cleaning helps interim.

- **Monitor Humidity Levels:** Use a hygrometer year-round; adjust dehumidifiers seasonally (higher in summer).

- **Check Walls and Ceilings:** Look for cracks, wet spots, or discoloration quarterly. Probe with a moisture meter if suspicious.

Your Journey to Recovery

Recovering from mold exposure is a personal journey that is different for everyone. It's about taking back your home and health one step at a time. Although mold can seem like an unseen enemy—persistent and sneaky—it is not insurmountable. Countless individuals have dramatically improved their lives by using the knowledge found in this guide. You too possess that capacity. Every step you take to create a mold-free or low-mold home puts you one step closer to wellness, whether you're fighting exhaustion, respiratory problems, or the fear of an invisible danger.

> **Tip:**
> Have your teen empty gym bags daily—mold festers in damp gear!

Progress, not perfection, is the goal of recovery. Start where you are: Schedule a mold inspection, get a hygrometer to track humidity, or open windows daily to air out your home. Little triumphs add up to dramatic change. Controlling moisture is the most effective strategy to prevent mold, according to the CDC, and every effort you make strengthens that foundation.

Your future does not have to be defined by the effects of mold. According to research from the National Institute of Environmental Health Sciences (NIEHS), lowering exposure over time can greatly alleviate symptoms, particularly when combined with supportive care. This guide and the larger community of survivors and specialists are here to support you. You are not alone on this journey. Celebrate your victories, have faith in your ability to feel better, and believe that recovery is possible.

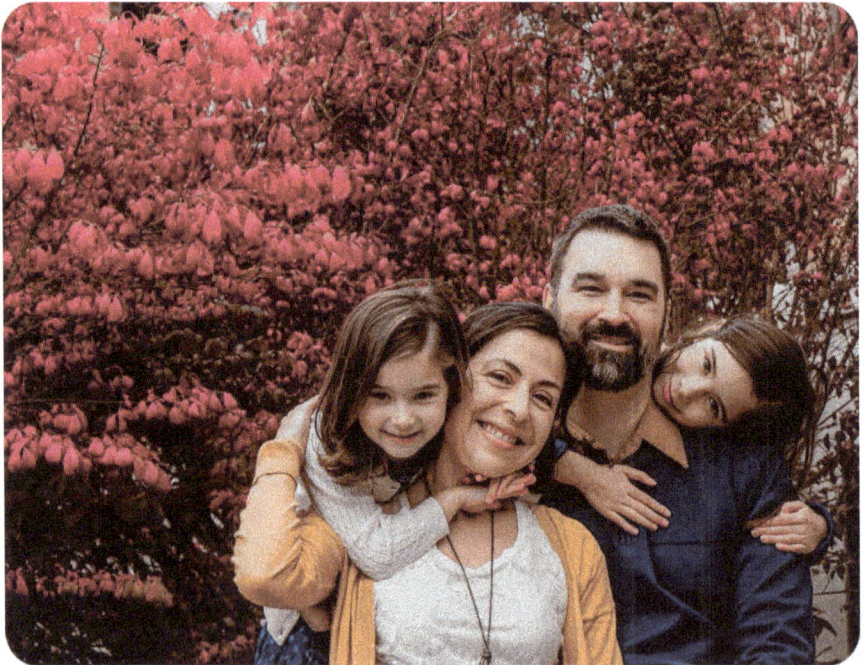

Triumph Over Mold: 5 Personal Recovery Stories

Case Study 1: The Teacher's Recovery

Patient Profile: Sarah M., 34-year-old elementary school teacher.
Exposure Duration: 2 years in a water-damaged classroom.

Initial Symptoms:

- Chronic fatigue

- Recurring sinus infections

- Brain fog and difficulty concentrating

- Persistent cough

- Unexplained anxiety

Recovery Journey:

1. **Initial Steps**

    a. Discovered black mold behind classroom walls

    b. Immediately relocated to different building

    c. Found temporary housing while remediating home

2. **Medical Intervention**

    a. Worked with environmental medicine specialist

    b. Comprehensive testing revealed elevated inflammatory markers

    c. Diagnosed with Chronic Inflammatory Response Syndrome (CIRS)

3. **Treatment Protocol**

    a. Binders to remove mycotoxins

    b. Antifungal nasal sprays

    c. Regular glutathione treatments

    d. Anti-inflammatory diet

    e. Air purification systems at home

> **Myth:**
> Bread is okay to eat if you remove the moldy piece.
>
> **Fact:**
> Mold threads weave through soft, porous bread—cutting it off won't help; mycotoxins might already be in the loaf, so toss it all.

Timeline and Outcome:

- Significant improvement after 6 months

- Full recovery at 18 months

- Currently advocates for classroom air quality

- Maintains preventive protocols

Case Study 2: The Young Athlete

Patient Profile: Marcus R., 19-year-old college swimmer.
Exposure Duration: 1 year in moldy dorm room.

Initial Symptoms:

- Declining athletic performance

- Shortness of breath

- Muscle weakness

- Joint pain

- Frequent headaches

Recovery Journey:

1. **Discovery and Action**

   a. Performance decline led to medical investigation

   b. Found significant mold growth in dorm ventilation

   c. Moved to new housing immediately

2. **Treatment Approach**

   a. Sports medicine specialist collaboration

   b. Respiratory therapy

   c. Detoxification protocols

   d. Strength rebuilding program

   e. Nutritional support

3. **Recovery Protocol**

   a. Specialized breathing exercises

   b. Gradual return to training

   c. Immune system support

   d. Regular sauna sessions

   e. Supplementation program

Timeline and Outcome:

- Return to training at 3 months
- Competition ready at 8 months
- Now performs at pre-exposure levels
- Advocates for athlete housing conditions

Case Study 3: The Remote Worker

Patient Profile: Jennifer L., 42-year-old software developer.
Exposure Duration: 3 years in the home office.

Initial Symptoms:

- Severe cognitive difficulties

- Memory problems

- Vision changes

- Chronic digestive issues

- Depression and mood swings

Tip: Add 5-10 drops of thyme or eucalyptus essential oil to laundry detergent!

Recovery Journey:

1. **Initial Steps**

    a. Home inspection revealed hidden bathroom leak

    b. Temporarily relocated during remediation

    c. Complete home office renovation

2. **Medical Support**

    a. Functional medicine approach

    b. Comprehensive neurological testing

    c. Gut health restoration protocol

    d. Mental health support

3. **Healing Protocol**

    a. Mycotoxin binding supplements

    b. Cognitive rehabilitation exercises

    c. Dietary modifications

    d. Stress reduction techniques

    e. Regular exercise program

Timeline and Outcome:

- Cognitive improvement at 4 months

- Substantial recovery at 12 months

- Now works as patient advocate

- Maintains strict home maintenance

Case Study 4: The Young Family

Patient Profile: The Wilson Family (Parents and 2 children under 10).
Exposure Duration: 18 months in a newly purchased home.

Initial Symptoms:

- Children: Recurring respiratory infections, rashes

- Parents: Fatigue, headaches, mood changes

- Family dog showing similar symptoms

Recovery Journey:

1. **Family Approach**

    a. Discovered hidden mold during renovation

    b. Whole family relocated temporarily

    c. Comprehensive family health evaluation

2. **Treatment Strategy**

   a. Pediatric environmental health specialist

   b. Family counseling support

   c. Individual treatment plans

   d. Pet veterinary care

3. **Recovery Methods**

   a. Child-appropriate detox protocols

   b. Family dietary changes

   c. Environmental modification

   d. Regular health monitoring

   e. Air quality management

Timeline and Outcome:

- Children recovered within 4 months

- Parents improved by 9 months

- Family now educates others

- Regular home testing protocol

Case Study 5: The Retiree

Patient Profile: Robert K., 68-year-old retired engineer.
Exposure Duration: 4 years in the affected retirement community.

Initial Symptoms:

- Balance problems

- Tremors
- Memory loss
- Sleep disturbances
- Respiratory issues

Recovery Journey:

1. **Initial Response**

     a. Symptoms initially misdiagnosed as age-related

     b. Environmental testing revealed mold

     c. Relocated to mold-free apartment

2. **Medical Intervention**

     a. Integrative medicine team

     b. Neurological rehabilitation

     c. Balance therapy

     d. Sleep study and treatment

     e. Respiratory support

3. **Recovery Protocol**

     a. Targeted supplementation

     b. Physical therapy

     c. Cognitive exercises

     d. Regular detoxification

     e. Air quality management

Timeline and Outcome:

- Initial improvement at 3 months
- Significant recovery at 12 months
- Now leads senior health group
- Maintains prevention protocol

Key Recovery Patterns Observed:

1. Early recognition and removal from exposure is crucial
2. Multi-faceted treatment approaches work best
3. Patient education plays vital role
4. Support systems aid recovery
5. Prevention protocols prevent relapse
6. Regular monitoring ensures continued health
7. Recovery timelines vary significantly
8. Lifestyle modifications support healing

Common Success Factors:

1. Prompt removal from exposure
2. Comprehensive medical support
3. Patient commitment to protocol
4. Environmental modification
5. Ongoing maintenance practices

6. Regular health monitoring

7. Support system engagement

8. Lifestyle adaptations

Prevention Recommendations:

1. Regular home inspections

2. Prompt moisture control

3. Air quality monitoring

4. Quick response to water damage

5. Regular maintenance

6. Air purification

7. Environmental testing

8. Health awareness

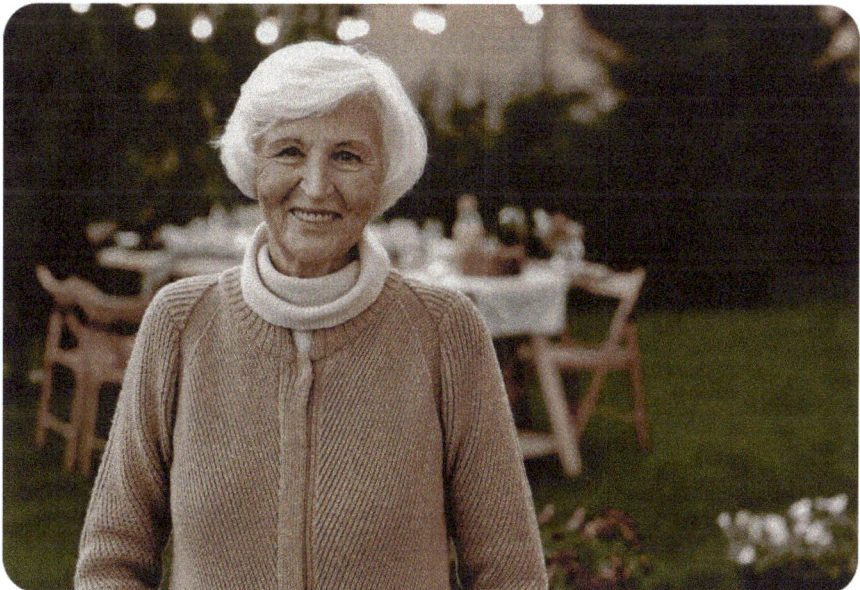

Mold Building Nightmares: 10 Real-Life Lessons

Case Study 1: Historic Library Recovery

Location: Boston, Massachusetts
Setting: 19th-century public library building
Problem: Water damage from burst pipe in winter led to extensive mold growth in basement archives

Situation:

- Burst pipe went unnoticed for 48 hours during holiday closure

- Affected 3,000 square feet of basement storage

- Rare books and documents exposed to high moisture

- Visible mold growth on walls, shelving, and materials

Solution:

- Immediate implementation of climate control measures

- Installation of industrial dehumidifiers

- Document preservation specialists brought in

- HEPA filtration system installed

- Materials individually assessed and treated

- Some documents required freeze-drying

Outcome:

- 85% of materials saved

- New moisture detection system installed

- Emergency response plan created

- Regular staff training implemented

References

1. Katz, A. (2014, March 7). Breaking Out of the Library Mold, in Boston and Beyond. *The New York Times*. Retrieved from https://www.nytimes.com/2014/03/08/us/breaking-out-of-the-library-mold-in-boston-and-beyond.html

2. PowerBees. (2016, September 16). Mold Threatens Boston Library Rare Books. Retrieved from https://www.powerbees.com/blog/mold-threatens-boston-library-rare-books

3. U.S. Environmental Protection Agency. (2024, March 5). A Brief Guide to Mold, Moisture, and Your Home. Retrieved from https://www.epa.gov/mold/brief-guide-mold-moisture-and-your-home

> **Tip:** Check fridge seals and drip pans—mold's sneaky hideout!

Case Study 2: Apartment Complex Post-Hurricane

Location: Miami, Florida
Setting: 200-unit apartment complex
Problem: Hurricane flooding led to widespread mold growth across multiple floors

Situation:

- Storm surge flooded first two floors

- Power outage lasted 5 days

- High humidity and heat accelerated mold growth

- 50 units severely affected

Solution:

- Building-wide assessment conducted

- Staged evacuation of affected units

- Complete removal of affected drywall and insulation

- Installation of commercial drying equipment

- Anti-microbial treatments applied

- HVAC system cleaning and sanitization

Outcome:

- Residents returned after 6 weeks

- Insurance covered majority of costs

- Building code updates implemented

- New flood prevention measures installed

References

1. WPTV News Staff. (2023, September 7). Mold cases grow in Palm Beach County during humid, stormy summer. *WPTV News*. Retrieved from https://www.wptv.com/news/local-news/investigations/mold-cases-grow-in-palm-beach-county-during-humid-stormy-summer

2. Davis, K. (2023, October 13). "A complete nightmare:" A gas leak, mold and delayed repairs at the Cloisters. *The Miami Hurricane*. Retrieved from

Case Study 3: Elementary School Recovery

Location: Portland, Oregon
Setting: Public elementary school
Problem: Hidden roof leak led to extensive mold growth in ceiling and walls

Situation:

- Teachers reported respiratory issues

- Air quality tests revealed elevated spore counts

- Inspection found significant hidden mold

- Affected multiple classrooms

Solution:

- Summer break used for remediation

- Complete roof replacement

- Removal of all contaminated materials

- Installation of improved ventilation system

- Regular air quality monitoring implemented

- Staff health screening program established

Outcome:

- Zero mold-related incidents following year

- Improved indoor air quality

- New maintenance protocols established

- Regular inspections scheduled

References

1. OPB News Staff. (2024, February 2). Fungal spores in Portland's Creston Elementary causing smelly unsafe conditions for students and staff, report shows. *OPB News*. Retrieved from https://www.opb.org/article/2024/02/02/fungal-spores-in-portlands-creston-elementary-causing-smelly-unsafe-conditions-for-students-and-staff-report-shows/

2. National Institute of Environmental Health Sciences. (n.d.). Mold. Retrieved from https://www.niehs.nih.gov/health/topics/agents/mold

3. Education Week. (2001, November 1). Clearing The Air. *Education Week*. Retrieved from https://www.edweek.org/education/clearing-the-air/2001/11

Case Study 4: Clinic Room

Location: Chicago, Illinois
Setting: Major urban health clinic
Problem: Mold discovered in operating room HVAC system

Situation:

- Routine inspection revealed mold in ductwork

- Potential exposure risk to patients

- Required immediate action

Solution:

- Emergency shutdown of affected areas

- Complete HVAC system cleaning

- Installation of UV-C light systems

- Implementation of new filtration standards

- Daily monitoring protocol established

- Staff training on early detection

Outcome:

- Zero patient infections reported

- Enhanced air quality standards met

- New preventive maintenance schedule

- Regular testing protocol implemented

References

1. CBS News. (2019, July 3). Seattle Children's Hospital mold infections leave one dead, force shutdown of operating rooms. Retrieved from https://www.cbsnews.com/news/seattle-childrens-hospital-mold-death-shutdown-most-operating-rooms-delaying-surgeries-2019-07-03/

2. Pereira, M. (2014, November 15). Mold contamination in a controlled hospital environment: a 3-year surveillance study. *PMC*. Retrieved from https://pmc.ncbi.nlm.nih.gov/articles/PMC4236478/

3. ResearchGate. (n.d.). Mold remediation in a hospital. Retrieved from

Case Study 5: Food Processing Facility

Location: Sacramento, California
Setting: Commercial bakery
Problem: Mold contamination in production area

Tip:
Toss old sponges—mold hides in the pores!

Situation:

- Regular testing revealed elevated spore counts

- Production had to be halted

- FDA inspection pending

- Employee health concerns

Solution:

- Complete facility shutdown for 72 hours

- Deep cleaning of all surfaces

- Update of humidity control systems

- Implementation of new sanitation protocols

- Employee training program

- Installation of air quality monitoring system

Outcome:

- Passed FDA inspection

- Zero product contamination

- Improved employee satisfaction

- Enhanced safety protocols

References

1. AOL News. (2024, July 26). Mold, grease and 'potentially hazardous' food: See Sacramento County health inspection results. Retrieved from https://www.aol.com/mold-grease-potentially-hazardous-food-120000731.html

Case Study 6: Historic Theater Renovation

Location: New Orleans, Louisiana
Setting: 1920s theater building
Problem: Long-term water intrusion led to extensive mold damage

Situation:

- Building vacant for 5 years

- Severe moisture problems throughout

- Historical preservation requirements

- Structural integrity concerns

Solution:

- Collaborative approach with preservation experts

- Custom remediation protocols developed

- Selective material replacement

- Modern moisture control systems added

- Original features preserved where possible

- New drainage systems installed

Outcome:

- Successfully preserved 80% of original features

- Modern safety standards met

- Reopened as functional theater

- Regular maintenance program established

References

1. WWLTV News. (2024, August 22). Resurrected, century-old theater in Bywater seeks help for repairs. Retrieved from https://www.wwltv.com/article/news/local/new-orleans-resurrected-century-old-theater-in-bywater-seeks-help-for-repairs/289-18d3b1e1-4ef4-4d25-a3ee-76c11cfa2a4c

Case Study 7: University Dormitory

Location: Seattle, Washington
Setting: 400-bed student housing facility
Problem: Widespread mold growth due to inadequate ventilation

Situation:

- Multiple student health complaints

- Visible mold in bathrooms and closets

- Outdated ventilation system

- High occupancy rates

Solution:

- Phased remediation during summer break

- Installation of new ventilation system

- Bathroom renovations

- Dehumidification systems added

- Student education program

- Regular inspection schedule

Outcome:

- 90% reduction in moisture-related complaints

- Improved student satisfaction

- Lower maintenance costs

- Enhanced building performance

References

1. Harris, K. (2022, April 22). In rainy Washington state, weak laws squash tenants' rights to mold remediation. *WHYY*. Retrieved from https://whyy.org/segments/in-rainy-washington-state-weak-laws-squash-tenants-rights-to-mold-remediation/

2. Reddit User. (2021, November 19). Mold in my dorm. *Reddit*. Retrieved from https://www.reddit.com/r/udub/comments/qxtjig/mold_in_my_dorm/

3. Weiss, M. (2018, September 28). U-Md. continues dorm cleanup after mold woes force students to relocate. *The Washington Post*. Retrieved from https://www.washingtonpost.com/education/2018/09/28/u-md-continues-dorm-cleanup-after-mold-woes-force-students-relocate/

Case Study 8: Luxury Yacht Recovery

Location: San Diego, California
Setting: 120-foot private yacht
Problem: Mold growth throughout interior after extended storage

Situation:

- Vessel stored without proper ventilation

- All interior surfaces affected

- Expensive furnishings damaged

- Complex electronic systems exposed

Solution:

- Complete interior removal

- Custom dehumidification system installed

- Specialized cleaning of electronics

- New ventilation system designed

- Anti-microbial treatments applied

- Regular maintenance schedule created

Outcome:

- Full restoration achieved

- New storage protocols developed

- Improved ventilation system

- Enhanced monitoring capabilities

Case Study 9: Office Building Recovery

Location: Houston, Texas
Setting: 15-story commercial office building
Problem: Widespread mold growth after flooding

Situation:

- Lower 3 floors flooded

- 200,000 square feet affected

- Business interruption concerns

- Multiple tenant complaints

Solution:

- Phased remediation plan

- Temporary relocation of tenants

- Complete replacement of affected materials

- Installation of flood barriers

- New water detection systems

- Updated emergency response plan

Outcome:

- All tenants retained

- Insurance costs reduced

- Improved building resilience

- Enhanced safety measures

References

1. Action Restoration. (n.d.). Disaster Recovery in Houston, TX. Retrieved from https://action-restoration.com/service-area/disaster-recovery/houston-tx/

Case Study 10: Wine Cellar Restoration

Location: Napa Valley, California
Setting: Commercial wine storage facility
Problem: Mold contamination threatening valuable wine collection

Situation:

- Climate control system failure

- $2 million in wine at risk

- Historic building limitations

- Time-sensitive situation

Solution:

- Emergency climate stabilization

- Custom filtration system installed

- UV treatment implementation

- Bottle-by-bottle inspection

- New monitoring technology

- Staff training program

Outcome:

- 99% of collection saved

- New preservation standards

- Enhanced storage protocols

- Improved insurance coverage

Key Lessons Learned Across All Cases:

1. Early detection is crucial for minimizing damage

2. Professional assessment leads to better outcomes

3. Proper documentation aids insurance claims

4. Employee/occupant education is essential

5. Regular maintenance prevents recurrence

6. Modern monitoring systems provide valuable data

7. Custom solutions often required for unique situations

8. Follow-up monitoring ensures long-term success

Tip: Wash kids' stuffed toys monthly—dusty plush traps mold!

Your Mold Recovery Toolkit: Must-Have Resources

Equip yourself with essential tools, expert support, and reliable knowledge to tackle mold challenges. Below are curated resources to guide you.

Professional Help

Need expert backup? Here's how to find certified pros and health resources:

Find a Certified Mold Inspector
Hire pros to spot mold and plan remediation—worth it for peace of mind!

- **United States:** Seek professionals certified by the American Council for Accredited Certification (ACAC) or the Institute of Inspection, Cleaning and Restoration Certification (IICRC). Search by zip code for a Certified Microbial Investigator (CMI) or Mold Remediation Specialist at ACAC.live or IICRC.org. Costs: $300–$800, based on home size and testing needs.

- **Canada:** Look for inspectors certified by the National Association of Mold Professionals (NAMP) or Inspect4Mold (Canadian-based). Find pros at moldpro.org or inspect4mold.ca—search by province. Costs: CAD 350–900, depending on scope.

- **European Union:** Seek experts accredited by the European Confederation of Indoor Air Quality (ECIAQ) or local bodies (e.g., British Damage Management Association in the UK). Visit eciaq.org or bdma.org.uk for directories—filter by country. Costs: €250–700, varies by region.

Environmental Health Center Database
Connect with clinics tackling mold-related illnesses—holistic help awaits!

- **United States:** The National Treatment Centers for Environmental Disease (NTCED) lists clinics specializing in mycotoxin testing and recovery, like their flagship in Jesup, GA. Visit ntced.org for locations.

- **Canada:** Check the Canadian Society for Environmental Medicine (CSEM) at csem.ca for practitioners focused on mold and environmental health—search by province.

- **European Union:** The European Academy of Environmental Medicine (EUROPAEM) offers a directory of mold-aware doctors at europaem.eu—filter by country.

Indoor Air Quality Association (IAQA)
Find air quality and remediation experts—science-backed solutions!

- **Global:** IAQA-certified pros span the U.S., Canada, and parts of the EU. Search iaqa.org's directory by location—ensures clean air expertise.

Emergency Contacts
Get quick answers on mold and air risks—call these pros!

- **United States:**

    - Environmental Protection Agency (EPA): Call the Safe Drinking Water Hotline at 1-800-426-4791 for mold and water damage queries. Monday–Friday, 8:30 AM–4:30 PM ET.

    - Indoor Air Quality Helpline (NCHH): Dial 1-800-513-2947 for expert advice on mold risks. Operated by the National Center for Healthy Housing, Monday–Friday, 9 AM–5 PM ET.

- **Canada:** Contact Health Canada's Indoor Air Quality line at 1-866-225-0709—guidance on mold and health risks, Monday–Friday, 8 AM–8 PM ET.

- **European Union:** Reach the European Environment Agency (EEA) via email at info@eea.europa.eu—mold resources vary by country, response within 2-3 days.

Support Groups

- **Surviving Mold Community Forum**
  Join peer discussions at survivingmold.com/community, guided by Dr. Ritchie Shoemaker's team. Ideal for sharing experiences on Chronic Inflammatory Response Syndrome (CIRS) and recovery.

- **Facebook Groups**

  - Toxic Mold Support: A 10,000+ member community (search "Toxic Mold Support" on Facebook) offering practical tips, doctor referrals, and support. Moderated for reliability.

  - Mold Recovery Group: A smaller, active group (search "Mold Recovery Group") focusing on detox strategies and success stories for encouragement.

In-Depth Books on Mold-Related Health Solutions

- **Break The Mold** by Dr. Jill Crista
  A 2018 guide with practical, naturopathic strategies for mold recovery, covering detox, diet, and home solutions. Available on Amazon or drjillcrista.com.

- **Mold Controlled** by John C. Banta
  A clear guide to identifying, fixing, and preventing mold in homes, with advice on seeking professional help. Find it on Amazon.

- **Toxic** by Neil Nathan, MD
  Published in 2018, this book explores mold's systemic effects and integrative treatments like binders. Updated for 2025 trends, available on Amazon or neilnathanmd.com.

- **Mold Illness: Surviving and Thriving** by Paula Vetter, Laurie Rossi, Cindy Edwards (Foreword by Ritchie C. Shoemaker)
  A recovery manual for patients and families impacted by CIRS, offering actionable steps. Available on Amazon.

Additional Reading

- **EPA Guidelines on Mold Remediation**
  A free, evidence-based resource, "Mold Remediation in Schools and Commercial Buildings," updated in 2023 for moisture control. Download at epa.gov.

Database: Find a Mold-Literate Health Practitioner Near You

- Visit drcrista.com/doctor-finder/ for a directory of mold-savvy health professionals.

Bio-resonance Health Scans

- Visit https://www.bioresonancescans.com/ to learn how this technology can help you for this and for many other symptoms.

- Click here for a 10% discount on a full health scan. Write to info@bioresonancescans.com to book your introductory call.o@bioresonancescans.com

- Ready to reclaim your health? Click here to watch an inspiring talk on healing from chronic conditions such as fatigue, allergies, and pain—practical steps to feel better, starting now.

Top Podcasts to Deepen Mold Awareness and Prevention

Explore expert insights, practical tips, and research through these engaging podcasts, perfect for homeowners and health enthusiasts alike.

- **The Mould Show** with Dr. Cameron Jones
  Learn to manage indoor air quality and reduce mold toxins with host Dr. Cameron Jones, a mold expert. Weekly episodes feature practical advice and interviews. Listen at Apple Podcasts.

- **Mold Matters** with Mike Adams and Jeremy Evans
  Mold expert Mike Adams and health advocate Jeremy Evans explain mold sickness and remediation essentials. Available on Apple Podcasts.

- **The Toxic Mold Podcast** with Steve Worstley
  A homeowner's guide to understanding toxic mold, its health risks, and prevention strategies. Tune in at Apple Podcasts.

Shopping Guide for Mold-Safe Products

Recommendations for HEPA purifiers, dehumidifiers, and non-toxic cleaners.

Air Purifiers with HEPA Filtration

Premium Options
1. Alen BreatheSmart 75i

- **Coverage:** Up to 1,300 sq ft (2 air changes/hour)

- **Features:** True HEPA filter captures 99.97% of particles down to 0.3 microns, smart sensor adjusts to air quality

- **Benefits:** Medical-grade filtration removes mold spores, whisper-quiet (25-49 dB), ideal for severe sensitivities

- **Price Range:** $749-$849

- **Ideal For**: Large rooms, open spaces, homes with mold-sensitive individuals

2. IQAir HealthPro Plus

- **Coverage:** Up to 1,125 sq ft (2 air changes/hour)

- **Features:** HyperHEPA filter captures particles down to 0.003 microns, advanced gas and odor filtration

- **Benefits:** Traps ultra-fine mold spores and mycotoxins, long filter life (up to 4 years), Swiss-made precision

- **Price Range:** $899-$999

- **Ideal For:** Extreme mold sensitivity, compromised immune systems, high-mold environments

3. Austin Air HealthMate Plus

- **Coverage:** Up to 1,500 sq ft (2 air changes/hour)

- **Features:** 4-stage filtration with true medical-grade HEPA, 15 lbs of activated carbon/zeolite

- **Benefits:** Removes mold spores, VOCs, and mycotoxins, durable 5-year filter life, robust steel construction

- **Price Range:** $715-$845

- **Ideal For:** Chemical and mold sensitivity, comprehensive air cleaning in large areas

Mid-Range Options
1. Coway Airmega 400

- **Coverage:** Up to 1,560 sq ft (2 air changes/hour)

- **Features:** True HEPA filter with washable pre-filter, real-time air quality indicator

- **Benefits:** Captures mold spores efficiently, smart mode saves energy, sleek design for open spaces

- **Price Range:** $449-$549

- **Ideal For:** Open floor plans, energy-conscious households with mold concerns

2. Medify Air MA-40

- **Coverage:** Up to 840 sq ft (2 air changes/hour)

- **Features:** H13 True HEPA filter captures 99.9% of particles down to 0.1 microns

- **Benefits:** High-grade filtration for mold spores, lifetime warranty with filter subscription, quiet (46-66 dB)

- **Price Range:** $329-$379

- **Ideal For:** Bedrooms, offices, smaller living spaces prone to mold

3. Medify MA-40 with Optional UV-C

- **Coverage:** Up to 840 sq ft (2 air changes/hour)

- **Features:** H13 HEPA filter (99.9% capture down to 0.1 microns), optional ozone-free UV-C light (254 nm)

- **Benefits:** Neutralizes mold spores without ozone, medical-grade filtration, quiet operation for sensitive users

- **Price Range:** $250-$300

- **Ideal For:** Bedrooms, living rooms, homes with mold-sensitive individuals

- **Ozone Safety:** Low-voltage UV-C emits only at 254 nm, confirmed ozone-free by Medify and user reviews

Budget-Friendly Options

1. Levoit Core 400S

- **Coverage:** Up to 400 sq ft (4 air changes/hour)

- **Features:** True HEPA filter with activated carbon, app and voice control (Alexa/Google)

- **Benefits**: Removes mold spores and odors, ultra-quiet sleep mode (24 dB), smart features for ease

- **Price Range:** $189-$219

- **Ideal For:** Bedrooms, small apartments with mild mold issues

2. GermGuardian AC5000E (Updated Model)

- **Coverage:** Up to 193 sq ft (4 air changes/hour)

- **Features:** True HEPA filter (99.97% capture at 0.3 microns), ozone-free UV-C light (254 nm)

- **Benefits:** Kills mold spores safely, reduces allergens and odors, compact for targeted use

- **Price Range:** $120-$160

- **Ideal For:** Medium rooms, pet areas, allergy sufferers in mold-prone spaces

- **Ozone Safety:** Updated bulb design ensures no ozone emission, verified by Guardian Technologies

3. SilverOnyx True HEPA Air Purifier

- **Coverage:** Up to 500 sq ft (2 air changes/hour)

- **Features:** 5-stage filtration with True HEPA and activated carbon, 5-speed touch control

- **Benefits:** Captures mold spores and mycotoxins, ultra-quiet (25 dB), effective for pets and allergies

- **Price Range:** $129-$179

- **Ideal For:** Large rooms, bedrooms, homes with pets or mild mold concerns

4. Pure Enrichment PureZone Elite 4-in-1

- **Coverage:** Up to 200 sq ft (4 air changes/hour)

- **Features:** True HEPA filter (99.97% capture at 0.3 microns), ozone-free UV-C sanitizer (254 nm)

- **Benefits:** Safely kills mold spores and bacteria, compact and Energy Star certified, affordable mold defense

- **Price Range:** $100-$150

- **Ideal For:** Small spaces, bathrooms, pet areas with mold risks

- **Ozone Safety:** Coated UV-C bulb emits only at 254 nm, independently tested as ozone-free

Dehumidifiers
Whole-House Solutions

1. Santa Fe Compact 70

- **Capacity:** 70 pints/day (at 80°F, 60% RH)

- **Coverage:** Up to 2,500 sq ft

- **Features:** Auto-defrost for low temperatures (down to 40°F), MERV-8 filter, optional ducting

- **Benefits:** Removes mold-causing moisture efficiently, energy-saving design, commercial-grade durability

- **Price Range:** $1,295-$1,495

- **Ideal For:** Basements, crawl spaces, whole-house mold prevention

2. Aprilaire E100 Pro Dehumidifier

- **Capacity:** 100 pints/day (at 80°F, 60% RH)

- **Coverage:** Up to 5,500 sq ft

- **Features:** Auto-defrost (operates down to 40°F), interactive digital control, built-in ducting compatibility

- **Benefits:** Controls humidity to stop mold growth, integrates with HVAC, backed by 5-year warranty

- **Price Range:** $1,395-$1,595

- **Ideal For:** Larger homes, comprehensive mold defense with HVAC systems

Room Dehumidifiers
1. hOmeLabs 4,500 Sq. Ft Energy Star Dehumidifier

- **Capacity:** 50 pints/day (at 86°F, 80% RH)

- **Coverage:** Up to 4,500 sq ft (ideal for 1,500 sq ft with frequent use)

- **Features:** Auto shut-off, continuous drain option, built-in pump

- **Benefits:** Keeps mold-prone areas dry, Energy Star certified, quiet operation (45-50 dB)

- **Price Range:** $219-$269

- **Ideal For:** Living rooms, large basements, multi-room mold control

2. Frigidaire FFAD5033W1

- **Capacity:** 50 pints/day (at 86°F, 80% RH)

- **Coverage:** Up to 3,000 sq ft (optimal for 1,000-1,500 sq ft)

- **Features:** Digital humidity readout, washable filter, continuous drain option

- **Benefits:** Prevents mold with precise humidity control, Energy Star rated, trusted brand reliability

- **Price Range:** $229-$279

- **Ideal For:** Medium to large rooms, spaces with moderate mold risks

3. Waykar 40 Pint Dehumidifier

- **Capacity:** 40 pints/day (at 86°F, 80% RH)

- **Coverage:** Up to 2,000 sq ft (best for 800-1,000 sq ft)

- **Features:** Auto-defrost (works down to 41°F), built-in hygrometer, auto shut-off

- **Benefits:** Maintains mold-free humidity (30-50%), intelligent controls, compact and portable

Tip: Peroxide kills 90%—spray and wait 10 minutes!

- **Price Range:** $159-$199

- **Ideal For:** Apartments, bedrooms, smaller homes with dampness issues

Mold-Cleaning Solutions: Efficacy, Uses, and Safety

Choosing the right mold-cleaning solution is key to effectively stopping mold growth while keeping your environment safe. Below, we evaluate a range of cleaning methods—UV-C lighting, hydrogen peroxide, vinegar, natural solutions, and professional-grade products—based on their efficacy, best uses, pros, cons, and safety considerations. Each method has unique strengths, so you can select the best tool for your specific mold challenge. Always use protective gear (mask, gloves, goggles, old clothes you can disinfect later or throw away) and ensure good ventilation when cleaning mold.

UV-C Lighting (254 nm, Ozone-Free)

- **Efficacy:** Kills 99%+ of mold spores on exposed surfaces (per EPA studies), but doesn't penetrate porous materials due to line-of-sight limitation—shadows block its effect. UV-C at 254 nm disrupts mold DNA, achieving 99.9% kill rates for fungi like Aspergillus with 25 mJ/cm² exposure (Block, 2001).

- **Format:** Available in portable units, air purifiers, or HVAC systems (e.g., Medify MA-40 UV-C).

- **Price Range:** $50-$200 for units, depending on size and features.

- **Pros:** Kills spores without moisture, no residue or fumes, ideal for continuous air/water sanitization.

- **Cons:** Requires line-of-sight, can't penetrate porous materials, may degrade plastics/fabrics over time, higher upfront cost.

- **Best Uses:**

- Dry, delicate items like books/papers (preserves pages).

- HVAC/ductwork (kills airborne spores).

- Humidifiers (sanitizes water/mist).

- Toothbrush holders (quick surface sterilization).

- Air purifiers (ongoing mold spore control).

- **Safety Notes:** Use ozone-free models to avoid respiratory irritation; wear protective glasses and avoid skin exposure during use.

- **Resources:**

  - U.S. Environmental Protection Agency (2024). "A Brief Guide to Mold, Moisture, and Your Home." epa.gov/mold/brief-guide-mold-moisture-and-your-home

  - International Ultraviolet Association (IUVA) (2021). "UV-C Disinfection Fact Sheet."

  - Block, S. S. (2001). Disinfection, Sterilization, and Preservation.

Hydrogen Peroxide (3%)

- **Efficacy:** Kills up to 90% of mold species on contact, oxidizing spores and mycotoxins (Springston et al., 2017). Achieves 85-95% reduction on hard surfaces like tile within 10-30 minutes, but efficacy drops on porous materials or against resistant species (e.g., Stachybotrys).

- **Format:** Available as pre-diluted 3% solution or food-grade 35% concentrate (dilute to 3% by mixing 1 part

35% hydrogen peroxide with 11 parts water, e.g., 1 oz + 11 oz water).

- **Price Range:** $2-$6 per quart (3% pre-diluted), $10-$30 per quart (35% concentrate).

- **Pros:** Safe for food-contact surfaces, penetrates porous materials, affordable, leaves no harmful residue, bleach-free.

- **Cons:** Requires moisture application (can damage paper), needs drying time, mild bleaching risk on fabrics, temporary effect (no residual protection).

- **Best Uses:**

  o Wet areas like hot tubs, pet bowls, drains.

  o Porous surfaces like carpets, mattresses, drywall.

  o Hard surfaces like tile, glass, appliances (e.g., fridge drip pans).

  o Spot treatments on bath toys, grout, non-porous items.

  o General cleaning of sinks, showers.

- **Safety Notes:** Safe at 3%, but store away from heat; higher concentrations (e.g., 35%) require careful dilution and gloves.

- **Resources:**

  o CDC (2023). "Mold Cleanup in Your Home." cdc.gov/mold/cleanup.htm

  - Springston, J. P., et al. (2017). "Efficacy of Hydrogen Peroxide on Mold Spores." Journal of Occupational and Environmental Hygiene.

Distilled White Vinegar (5-8%)

- **Efficacy:** Kills 82% of common mold species (e.g., Penicillium, Aspergillus) on contact due to its natural acidity, but less effective against tougher species like black mold (Stachybotrys) (Munk et al., 2001). Best for surface cleaning, not deep penetration.

- **Format:** Use standard household distilled white vinegar (5-8% acetic acid) straight from the bottle for maximum effectiveness, or dilute 1:1 with water (e.g., 8 oz vinegar + 8 oz water) for a spray. Stronger cleaning vinegar (6-8% acidity) may work slightly better but isn't necessary for minor mold issues.

- **Price Range:** $2-$5 per gallon.

- **Pros:** Non-toxic, very cheap, widely available, dissolves mold naturally.

- **Cons:** Less effective than peroxide (82% vs. 90%), strong odor, no residual prevention, may not tackle deep mold.

- **Best Uses:**

    - Maintenance in showers, windows.

    - Fabrics like towels, curtains.

    - Hard surfaces like countertops, tiles.

    - Minor surface mold spots.

    - DIY mixes with borax or peroxide.

- **Usage Tips:** Use undiluted for maximum effect; let sit on the moldy surface for at least an hour before wiping; repeated applications may be needed for stubborn mold or porous surfaces.

- **Safety Notes:** Safe, but avoid mixing with bleach (creates toxic chlorine gas); ventilate due to odor. (It's preferable to avoid bleach altogether due to its high toxicity.)

- **Resources:**

    o Munk, J., et al. (2001). "Antifungal Activity of Acetic Acid." Journal of Applied Microbiology.

    o Rutgers University Extension (2019). "Vinegar as a Disinfectant."

Natural Cleaning Solutions

Efficacy: Varies—Benefect (thymol) achieves near 99% on surfaces; essential oils hit 70-95% for mild cases; borax is effective as a preventative but less studied for direct mold killing (Nazzaro et al., 2013; Hammer et al., 2015).

Benefect Botanical Decon 30

- **Format:** Ready-to-use spray (32 oz) or gallon.

- **Active Ingredients:** Thymol (0.23%, derived from thyme oil).

- **Benefits:** 100% botanical, EPA-registered to kill mold and bacteria (99%+ pathogen kill, per Benefect claims), non-toxic with no synthetic chemicals.

- **Price Range:** $15-$25 (32 oz), $45-$55 (1 gallon).

- **Best Uses:** Food-contact surfaces, children's rooms, general mold-safe cleaning.

Moldex Mold Killer

- **Format:** Ready-to-use spray (32 oz).

- **Active Ingredients:** Hydrogen peroxide (3% stabilized solution).

- **Benefits:** EPA-registered mold killer, bleach-free, safe for regular use.

- Price Range: $9-$15.

- **Best Uses:** Bathrooms, hard surfaces (e.g., tile, glass), small mold outbreaks.

Borax

- **Format:** Powder (4-5 lb box).

- **Active Ingredients:** Sodium tetraborate decahydrate (natural mineral).

- **Benefits:** Natural antifungal cleaner, prevents mold regrowth, versatile for DIY solutions.

- **Price Range:** $5-$10.

- **Best Uses:** DIY mold-cleaning mixes, laundry additives to stop mold spores.

Tea Tree Oil

- **Format:** 1 tsp (5 mL) per cup (8 oz) of water as a spray solution.

- **Benefits:** Natural fungicide, pleasant earthy scent, safe for small-scale use.

- **Price Range:** $10-$20 per 1 oz bottle.

- **Best Uses:** Small mold spot treatments, aromatic cleaner for damp areas, mold prevention on surfaces.

- **Pros:** Botanical/eco-friendly, multi-purpose (e.g., borax for laundry), some EPA-registered (e.g., Benefect), pleasant scents (e.g., tea tree).

- **Cons:** Variable efficacy (e.g., tea tree less potent), higher cost than vinegar/peroxide, requires dilution (e.g., tea tree oil), limited penetration for deep mold.

- **Safety Notes:** Tea tree oil may irritate skin—test first; borax is mildly toxic if ingested, keep from pets/kids.

- **Resources:**

    - Benefect Product Data (2024). benefect.com (EPA Reg. No. 84683-1).

    - Nazzaro, F., et al. (2013). "Essential Oils and Antifungal Activity." Molecules.

    - Hammer, K. A., et al. (2015). "Antifungal Effects of Melaleuca Alternifolia." Journal of Applied Microbiology.

Thyme Oil

- **Format:** 1 tsp (5 mL) per cup (8 oz) of water as a spray solution.

- **Benefits:** Potent natural fungicide (90% inhibition of Candida and molds at 0.5% concentration), warm herbal scent, effective for small-scale mold control.

- **Price Range:** $12-$25 per 1 oz bottle.

- **Uses:** Small mold spot treatments, laundry odor eliminator, bathroom surface cleaner.

- **Pros:** Eco-friendly, multi-purpose (e.g., laundry boost), strong antifungal action per 2013 Journal of Medical Microbiology.

- **Cons:** Variable potency depending on thymol content, higher cost than vinegar, requires dilution.

- **Safety Notes:** May irritate skin—test first; avoid ingestion, keep away from pets/kids.

- **Resources:**

  - Nazzaro, F., et al. (2013). "Essential Oils and Antifungal Activity." Molecules.

  - Odds, F. C., et al. (2013). "Thyme Oil Inhibitory Effects." Journal of Medical Microbiology.

Clove Oil

- **Format:** 1 tsp (5 mL) per cup (8 oz) of water as a spray solution.

- **Benefits:** Powerful antifungal (85% reduction of Aspergillus at 0.4% concentration), spicy aroma, wood-safe mold prevention.

- **Price Range:** $10-$22 per 1 oz bottle.

- **Best Uses:** Shower curtain cleaner, wood surface treatment, musty clothing refresher.

- **Pros:** Botanical and effective, multi-use (e.g., grout cleaner), backed by International Journal of Food Microbiology (2007).

- **Cons:** Strong scent may linger, more expensive than peroxide, needs dilution.

- **Safety Notes:** Eugenol may cause skin irritation—patch test; keep out of reach of children/pets.

- **Resources:**

    - Pinto, E., et al. (2007). "Antifungal Activity of Clove Oil." International Journal of Food Microbiology.

Oregano Oil

- **Format:** 0.5 tsp (2.5 mL) per cup (8 oz) of water as a spray solution.

- **Benefits:** Exceptional fungicide (95% inhibition of Penicillium at 0.25% concentration), robust earthy scent, ideal for odor control.

- **Price Range:** $15-$30 per 1 oz bottle.

- **Best Uses:** Outdoor spaces around the home and garden, mattress refresher, gym bag cleaner, laundry odor neutralizer.

- **Pros:** Highly potent per Journal of Food Protection (2001), eco-friendly, versatile.

- **Cons:** Intense aroma, higher cost, requires careful dilution.

- **Safety Notes:** Carvacrol may irritate skin—test first; store safely.

- **Resources:**

    - Lambert, R. J. W., et al. (2001). "Oregano Oil Antifungal Effects." Journal of Food Protection.

Eucalyptus Oil

- **Format:** 1 tsp (5 mL) per cup (8 oz) of water as a spray solution.

- **Benefits:** Effective mold inhibitor (70% reduction of Alternaria at 1% concentration), fresh minty scent, great for damp spaces.

- **Price Range:** $8-$18 per 1 oz bottle.

- **Best Uses:** Towel odor prevention, closet spray, fabric refresher.

- **Pros:** Pleasant aroma, eco-friendly, supported by Mycopathologia (2010).

- **Cons:** Less potent than oregano/thyme, limited deep mold penetration, needs dilution.

- **Safety Notes:** May cause mild skin irritation—test first; keep away from pets/kids.

- **Resources:**

  - Cimanga, K., et al. (2010). "Eucalyptus Oil Antifungal Properties." Mycopathologia.

Cinnamon Oil

- **Format:** 0.75 tsp (3.75 mL) per cup (8 oz) of water as a spray solution.

- **Benefits:** Strong antifungal (80% inhibition of Aspergillus at 0.3% concentration), warm spicy scent, excellent for stubborn molds.

- **Price Range:** $12-$25 per 1 oz bottle.

- **Best Uses:** Shoe storage spray, basement cleaner, laundry boost for musty items.

- **Pros:** Botanical, multi-purpose, validated by Journal of Antimicrobial Chemotherapy (2006).

- **Cons:** Potent aroma may overwhelm, higher cost, requires dilution.

- **Safety Notes:** Cinnamaldehyde may irritate skin—test first; store securely from pets/kids.

- **Resources:**

  - Simić, A., et al. (2006). "Cinnamon Oil Antifungal Activity." Journal of Antimicrobial Chemotherapy.

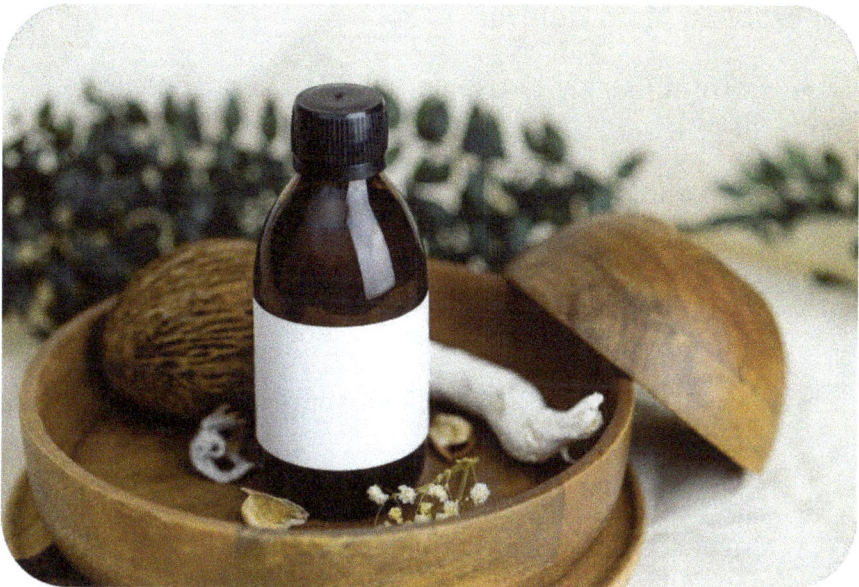

Professional-Grade Solutions

Efficacy: Kills 95-99.99% of mold and pathogens, often lab-tested and hospital-grade (e.g., BenzaRid achieves 99.99%,

Concrobium 95-98%). Outperforms natural options due to stronger formulations.

EC3 Mold Solution Concentrate

- **Format:** Liquid concentrate (16 oz makes 1 gallon).

- **Active Ingredients:** Citrus seed extracts, natural botanical extracts.

- **Benefits:** Non-toxic mold killer, safe for sensitive users, lab-tested to reduce mold counts.

- **Price Range:** $29-$35.

- **Best Uses:** Treating visible mold on surfaces, preventative HVAC maintenance, laundry additive.

Concrobium Mold Control

- **Format:** Ready-to-use spray (32 oz) or concentrate (1 gallon).

- **Active Ingredients:** Sodium carbonate, trisodium phosphate, proprietary inorganic compounds.

- **Benefits:** EPA-registered to kill and prevent mold growth, bleach-free, leaves protective barrier.

- **Price Range:** $13-$20 (32 oz spray), $30-$40 (1 gallon concentrate).

- **Best Uses:** Hard surfaces (e.g., tile, drywall), fabrics, crawl spaces, prevention (barrier).

BenzaRid

- **Format:** Liquid concentrate (32 oz makes 2 gallons).

- **Active Ingredients:** Thymol, quaternary ammonium compounds, botanical extracts.

- **Benefits:** Hospital-grade, odorless, non-staining.

- **Price Range:** $39-$49.

- **Best Uses:** Post-remediation cleanup, regular mold maintenance on non-porous surfaces, severe mold cases.

- **Pros:** High efficacy, EPA-registered (e.g., Concrobium, BenzaRid), residual protection (e.g., Concrobium barrier), hospital-grade options.

- **Cons:** More expensive than natural options, stronger chemicals (e.g., BenzaRid), may require safety gear (e.g., gloves).

- **Safety Notes:** Check labels—some (e.g., BenzaRid) suggest masks/ventilation during use.

- **Resources:**

  - BenzaRid Product Data (2024). benzrid.com (EPA Reg. No. 10324-85).

  - Concrobium Product Data (2024). concrobium.com (EPA Reg. No. 82552-1).

  - EPA (2023). "List N: Disinfectants for Use Against Mold."

Note: While these products are scientifically proven to have antifungal properties, they are not a complete replacement for addressing underlying moisture issues or extensive mold infestations. For significant mold problems, consult professional remediation services.

Tip: Add flax to your lunch—detox starts today!

Tools for Mold Detection, Prevention, and Safe Cleanup

Detecting and cleaning up mold requires the right tools—from testing kits to identify mold growth, to moisture meters and humidity monitors to prevent it, to protective gear for safe removal. This section equips you with everything you need to tackle mold effectively, whether you're assessing your home, monitoring for future risks, or performing a DIY cleanup. We've also included trusted retailers to help you source high-quality products, ensuring you can stop mold in its tracks and create a healthier environment for you and your loved ones.

Mold Testing Kits

- **ImmunoLytics Mold Test Kit**

    o Type: Petri dish culture test (swab or plate options).

    o Benefits: Easy-to-use for beginners, includes lab analysis with detailed mold species identification.

    o Price Range: $30-$45 per test (includes lab fee).

    o Best For: Initial mold assessment, verifying post-remediation success.

- **Mold Armor Do It Yourself Mold Test Kit**

    o Type: Surface swab and optional air sampling (petri dish).

    o Benefits: Affordable, fast surface results in 48 hours, no lab fee for basic testing.

    o Price Range: $8-$15.

- Best For: Quick preliminary mold checks, DIY home assessments.

- **My Mold Detective MMD103 Mold Test Kit**

  - Type: Air sampling system with reusable pump.

  - Benefits: Professional-grade air spore capture, lab analysis included, reusable pump for multiple tests.

  - Price Range: $59-$79 (starter kit with 1 sample), $20-$30 (additional samples).

  - Best For: Comprehensive home air testing, detecting hidden mold sources.

Moisture Meters and Humidity Monitors

- **Protimeter BLD5365 Surveymaster**

  - Type: Dual-function moisture meter.

  - Features: Pin and pinless moisture detection, built-in hygrometer.

  - Benefits: Professional-grade, detects hidden moisture in materials.

  - Price Range: $495-$595.

  - Best For: Serious mold investigators, homeowners after water damage.

- **General Tools MMD4E Digital Moisture Meter**

  - Type: Pin-type moisture meter.

  - Features: LED display, audible alert, multiple material settings.

- Benefits: Accurate readings in wood, drywall, and other building materials.

- Price Range: $35-$45.

- Best For: Finding potential moisture problems before mold develops.

- **Govee Indoor Hygrometer Thermometer**

  - Type: Digital humidity monitor.

  - Features: Bluetooth connection, data logging, alerts.

  - Benefits: Affordable, easy to use, ideal for multiple room monitoring.

  - Price Range: $15-$25.

  - Best For: Regular humidity monitoring to prevent mold growth.

Protective Gear for DIY Mold Cleanup

- 3M 8511 N95 Respirator

  - Type: Disposable respirator mask.

  - Features: Exhalation valve, adjustable nose clip.

  - Benefits: Filters 95% of airborne particles.

  - Price Range: $20-$30 (10-pack).

  - Best For: Small cleanup jobs, light exposure.

- **3M 6800 Full Face Respirator**

  - Type: Reusable full-face respirator.

- Features: Wide field of vision, accepts various filters.

  - Benefits: Complete face protection, comfortable fit.

  - Price Range: $150-$180 (mask only), $50-$70 (P100 filters).

  - Best For: Serious mold remediation, professionals.

- **DuPont Tyvek Disposable Coveralls**

  - Type: Full-body protective suit.

  - Features: Hood, elastic wrists and ankles.

  - Benefits: Particle protection, tear-resistant.

  - Price Range: $8-$15 per suit.

  - Best For: Extensive mold cleanup, attic/crawlspace work.

Recommended Retailers

- Bulk Peroxide (https://bulkperoxide.com): Wide selection of high-quality hydrogen peroxide in varying strengths.

- Home Depot / Lowe's: Dehumidifiers, basic cleaning supplies, DIY materials.

- Amazon: Wide selection of all product categories, often at competitive prices.

Tip:
Vinegar-soak rags—wipe mold without spreading spores!

- MicroBalance Health Products (https://microbalancehealthproducts.com): Specializes in EC3 and other mold-specific products.

- AllergyBuyersClub.com: Curated selection of air purifiers for mold sensitivity.

- Sylvane.com: High-quality dehumidifiers and air quality products.

- Home Air Guides (https://homeairadvisor.com/air-purifiers): Educational resources plus product recommendations for air purifiers.

Everyday Mold Q&A: Practical Answers

1. Can I still use a cutting board if I spot mold on it?
Mold on a cutting board is a red flag—it's often a sign of trapped moisture and food residue.

- **Wooden Cutting Boards**: Mold can penetrate the porous surface, especially if the board has deep knife grooves. If the mold is light (small spots), scrub it with hot, soapy water, then soak in a solution of 1 tablespoon vinegar per cup of water with 5-10 drops of clove essential oil for 10 minutes. Rinse, dry thoroughly, and sand the surface lightly to remove any lingering spores. If the mold is extensive or deep, toss the board—spores can hide in the wood grain.

- **Plastic Cutting Boards**: Less porous, so mold is usually surface-level. Wash with hot, soapy water, then disinfect with a 3% hydrogen peroxide solution (apply directly, let sit for 5 minutes, then rinse). If the mold persists or the board is heavily scratched (a breeding ground for mold), replace it.

- **Prevention Tip**: Always dry cutting boards completely after washing, and store them upright to avoid trapping moisture.

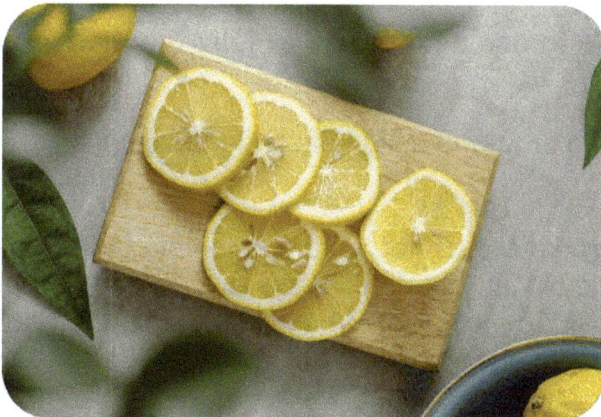

2. Can I eat fruit with mold on it if I cut off the moldy part?

Mold on fruit can be tricky—it often spreads deeper than you can see.

- **Firm Fruits (e.g., apples, pears):** If the mold is a small spot, you can cut away at least an inch around and below it. The rest might be safe to eat, but check for a musty smell or off taste—mold can leave behind mycotoxins that penetrate firm fruits slightly. When in doubt, toss it.

- **Soft Fruits (e.g., berries, peaches):** Toss the whole fruit. Mold spreads easily through soft, juicy textures, and even non-moldy parts can be contaminated with spores or toxins. If one berry in a pack is moldy, check the rest closely—spores spread fast.

- **Prevention Tip:** Store fruit in the fridge to slow mold growth, and don't let it sit in a damp fruit bowl. Wash and dry fruit before storing to remove surface spores.

- **Bonus Tip:** Brown spots on fruit indicate bacteria that create rot—and mold often follows. Always cut these out generously- no matter how small and insignificant they seem. Being proactive about how you handle, store, and prepare your food is an essential part of smart food hygiene and mindful eating.

3. Is it safe to use a jar of jam or jelly that has mold on the surface?

Mold on jam or jelly is a sign of spoilage, and it's not worth the risk.

- **Surface Mold:** You might be tempted to scoop off the moldy layer, but don't. Jams and jellies are soft and moist, so mold roots (mycelium) can penetrate deep, even if you remove an inch or more. Plus, some molds produce mycotoxins that can spread through the whole jar. Toss it.

- **Check Nearby Jars:** Mold spores can spread to other jars in your pantry, so inspect nearby items for signs of growth or a musty smell.

- **Storage Tip:** Always use a clean spoon to scoop jam—introducing crumbs or moisture can invite mold. Store opened jars in the fridge and use it up quickly.

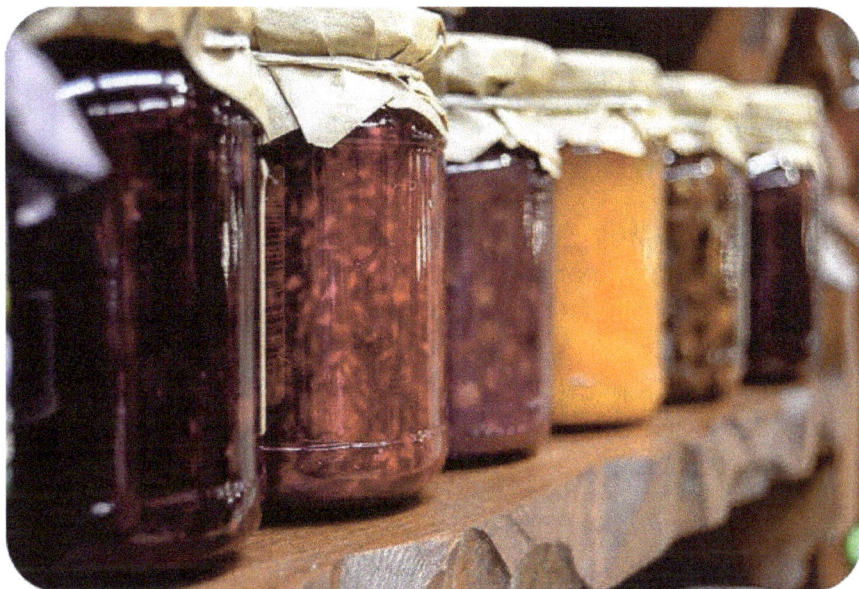

4. Is it safe to keep clothes that have a musty, moldy smell?

That musty smell often means mold or mildew has started growing on the fabric, especially if it was stored damp.

- **Light Odor:** Wash the clothes in hot water (if the fabric allows) with a cup of white vinegar added to the cycle along with 5-10 drops of clove, thyme, tea tree, or eucalyptus oil. Dry in direct sunlight if possible—UV light helps kill mold spores. Smell test after: if the odor's gone, they're likely safe.

- **Visible Mold or Persistent Smell:** Mold may have penetrated the fibers, especially on natural fabrics like cotton or wool. Machine wash with vinegar and a mold-killing detergent (like Benefect), but if the smell or spots remain, the mold might be too deep—consider discarding the item to avoid spreading spores.

- **Pro Tip:** Never store clothes in damp areas (like basements) without proper ventilation. Use silica gel packets or a dehumidifier to keep storage spaces dry.

5. What should I do if I find mold on my leather shoes or bag?

Leather is prone to mold in humid conditions, but you can often save it if you act fast.

- **Surface Mold:** Wipe the leather with a cloth dipped in a 1:1 mix of water and vinegar and 2-3 drops of clove essential oil. Avoid soaking—leather doesn't like too much moisture. Let it air dry completely, then apply a leather conditioner to prevent drying out.

- **Deep Mold (e.g., inside shoes):** If the mold has spread inside or the smell lingers, it's harder to fully remove. Use a vinegar solution to wipe down, stuff with newspaper to absorb moisture, and dry in a well-ventilated area. If the mold persists, professional cleaning might be needed—or it's time to toss.

- **Prevention:** Store leather goods in a dry, airy place. Avoid plastic bags—they trap moisture. Use cedar shoe inserts or silica packets to absorb humidity.

6. Can I eat bread if I cut off the moldy part?

Unlike hard cheese, bread is a no-go once mold appears.

- **Why It's Unsafe:** Bread is soft and porous, so mold roots (mycelium) spread deep beyond the visible spot, even if you cut away an inch or more. Some molds on bread can produce mycotoxins, which are harmful if ingested.

- **What to Do:** Toss the whole loaf, including any slices that might have been in contact. Check nearby food items—mold spores can spread easily in pantries.

- **Storage Tip:** Don't wrap it in a plastic bag and leave it out on the counter. Keep bread in a cool, dry place, and consider freezing if you don't eat it quickly. Mold loves warm, humid environments like your kitchen counter.

7. Is it okay to use a book or notebook with mold spots on the pages?

Mold on paper can be tricky—it's often a sign of water damage, and spores can spread.

- **Light Mold (Surface Spots):** Isolate the book in a sealed plastic bag to prevent spore spread. Brush off loose mold outdoors with a dry cloth (wear a mask!). Then, lightly mist the pages with a 1:1 water-vinegar solution, and let them air dry in sunlight. If the pages aren't too damaged, you can likely keep the book.

- **Heavy Mold or Musty Smell:** If the mold has penetrated deeply (pages sticking together, strong odor), it's usually not salvageable. Mold can degrade paper over time, and the spores might trigger allergies. Discard it, and check nearby books for spread.

- **Prevention:** Store books in a dry, well-ventilated area. Avoid stacking them tightly in humid spaces like basements.

8. What about mold on a wooden spoon or other kitchen utensils?

Wooden utensils are porous, so mold can be a problem if they're not dried properly.

- **Surface Mold:** Scrub with hot, soapy water, then soak in a vinegar and clove essential oil solution (1:1 water and vinegar 3-5 drops of clove essential oil) for 15 minutes. Rinse, dry thoroughly in sunlight, and lightly sand if needed. If the spoon looks clean and odor-free, it's likely safe to use.

- **Deep Mold or Cracks:** If the mold has seeped into cracks or the wood feels soft, toss it. Spores can linger in the grain, and you don't want that in your food.

- **Care Tip:** After washing wooden utensils, dry them immediately—don't let them sit wet. Oil them occasionally with food-safe mineral oil to seal the wood.

9. Can I still sleep on a mattress with a small mold spot?

Mold on a mattress is a health concern—spores can affect air quality while you sleep.

- **Small Surface Mold:** Vacuum the spot with a HEPA-filter vacuum to remove loose spores (do this outside if possible). Clean with a 1:1 water-vinegar solution, then dry thoroughly with a fan or in sunlight. Test for any lingering smell—if it's gone, you might be okay, but monitor for recurrence.

- **Widespread Mold or Odor:** If the mold has spread or you smell mustiness inside the mattress, it's best to replace it. Mattresses are thick and absorbent, so mold often grows deep inside where you can't clean it.

- **Prevention:** Use a mattress protector, keep your bedroom humidity below 50%, and ensure good airflow under the bed.

10. Is it safe to use a moldy yoga mat or exercise equipment?

Mold on exercise gear can irritate skin or lungs, especially during sweaty workouts.

- **Surface Mold:** Wipe down with a 1:1 water-vinegar solution with 2-3 drops of tea tree, eucalyptus or thyme essential oil, then disinfect with a mild hydrogen peroxide spray (3% solution). Let it air dry completely. If the mat is non-porous (like PVC), it's usually salvageable.

- **Porous Mats or Deep Mold:** If the mat is foam-based and the mold has penetrated (or it smells musty), replace it. Mold in porous materials can release spores when you move or sweat on it.

- **Pro Tip:** Roll up yoga mats only after they're fully dry, and store them in a ventilated area. Wipe down after each use to prevent moisture buildup.

11. Can I keep a rug or carpet with mold spots?

Mold on rugs or carpets can spread quickly, especially if they've been wet for a while.

- **Small Surface Mold:** Vacuum with a HEPA-filter vacuum to remove loose spores (do this outdoors if possible). Clean the spot with a 1:1 water-vinegar solution, scrub gently, and dry thoroughly with a fan or in sunlight. If the mold doesn't return and there's no smell, it's likely safe.

- **Deep Mold or Musty Odor:** If the mold has reached the backing or padding (or the rug smells musty even after cleaning), it's usually a lost cause. Mold spores can hide deep in fibers, and large rugs are hard to fully sanitize—consider professional cleaning or replacement.

- **Prevention:** Keep rugs dry, vacuum regularly, and avoid placing them in damp areas like basements without a dehumidifier.

12. Is it safe to use a refrigerator if I find mold inside?

Mold in a fridge isn't uncommon, especially in humid climates or if spills go unnoticed. It particularly likes to hide in the seals—the soft lining around the door and drip pans. Go look at your fridge now to see if you notice any black spots.

- **Light Mold**: Empty the fridge, wipe all surfaces with a 1:1 water-vinegar solution, and follow with a 3% hydrogen peroxide solution (wipe on, let sit for 5 minutes, then rinse). Dry thoroughly, then replace food. Check seals, drip pans, and corners—mold loves those spots. If it's clean and odor-free, it's fine to use.

- **Heavy Mold or Smell**: If mold has spread into cracks, insulation, or the drip pan (and cleaning doesn't remove the odor), it could keep coming back. You might need a deep clean by a pro or, in bad cases, a new fridge

- **Pro Tip**: Keep your fridge dry—wipe up spills immediately, and store food in sealed containers to limit moisture.

13. What do I do with a moldy backpack or luggage?

Mold on bags often comes from storing them wet or in humid spots.

- **Surface Mold:** Empty the bag, brush off loose mold outdoors (wear a mask), and wipe with a 1:1 water-vinegar solution with 5-10 drops of eucalyptus, clove, or thyme essential oil. For fabric, machine wash if the label allows; for leather or vinyl, air dry completely after wiping. If it's clean and odor-free, it's usable.

- **Deep Mold (e.g., in lining):** If the mold has penetrated stitching or inner layers and the smell lingers after cleaning, toss it. Spores can stick around and spread to what you pack next.

- **Prevention:** Dry bags fully before storing, and keep them in a ventilated area with silica gel packets to absorb humidity.

14. Can I still wear jewelry that's been in a moldy box?

Mold on jewelry itself is rare, but a moldy storage box can transfer spores or a musty smell.

- **Metal or Hard Surfaces:** Clean the jewelry with a cloth dipped in rubbing alcohol or a mild soap solution, then dry thoroughly. If there's no visible mold or odor, it's safe to wear.

- **Porous Materials** (e.g., wooden beads): If mold has grown on the jewelry itself, it's harder to clean fully. Try a vinegar wipe and dry in sunlight, but if the smell or spots persist, consider discarding. Clean the box too— vinegar or a UV-C light can help.

- **Storage Tip:** Store jewelry in a dry, sealed container with anti-humidity packets, not damp velvet boxes or basements.

15. Is it okay to use a car with mold on the seats or dashboard?

Mold in a car can come from spills, leaks, or high humidity— and it's a health risk if you're breathing it in.

- **Surface Mold:** Vacuum with a HEPA filter to remove spores (outside the car), then wipe seats or hard surfaces with a 1:1 water-vinegar solution. Dry with a fan or open windows in sunlight. If the mold's gone and there's no smell, it's fine to drive.

- **Deep Mold** (e.g., in upholstery): If mold has soaked into seats or carpet (or you smell it in the vents), it's tougher. Professional detailing might save it—otherwise, replacement parts or a new car might be your only fix.

- **Prevention:** Fix leaks ASAP and keep windows cracked in humid weather. If you park long-term, use a dehumidifier bag or pouch filled with a desiccant—like silica gel or calcium chloride—to absorb moisture

16. Can I eat cheese that has mold on it?

Mold on cheese isn't always harmful—it depends on the type of cheese and the mold.

- **Intentionally Moldy Cheeses (Safe)**: Some cheeses, like blue cheeses (e.g., Roquefort, Gorgonzola, Stilton) or soft-ripened cheeses (e.g., Brie, Camembert), are made with specific, safe molds like *Penicillium roqueforti* or *Penicillium camemberti*. These molds are carefully cultivated during the cheese-making process to develop flavor, texture, and character. They're not only harmless but essential to the cheese's identity. These molds don't produce harmful toxins under controlled conditions and are perfectly safe to eat.

- **Unintentional Mold on Cheese (Potentially Harmful)**: If mold grows on cheese that wasn't meant to have it—like cheddar, mozzarella, or a processed slice—it's usually a sign of spoilage. This mold could be a variety of species, some of which might produce mycotoxins or indicate contamination. While not all unplanned mold is dangerous, it's harder to tell what's safe without testing. The general advice is:

- *Hard Cheeses*: You can cut off the moldy part (at least an inch around and below it) and eat the rest, as mold doesn't penetrate deeply into dense cheese.

- *Soft Cheeses*: Toss it. Mold can spread more easily through softer, wetter textures, potentially contaminating the whole piece.

- **Why the Difference?** The molds used in cheese production are selected for their safety and beneficial properties, while wild molds that show up unexpectedly might not be. Factors like moisture, temperature, and the cheese's composition also affect whether mold becomes a problem. If you've got a specific cheese in mind, let me know, and I can dig deeper!

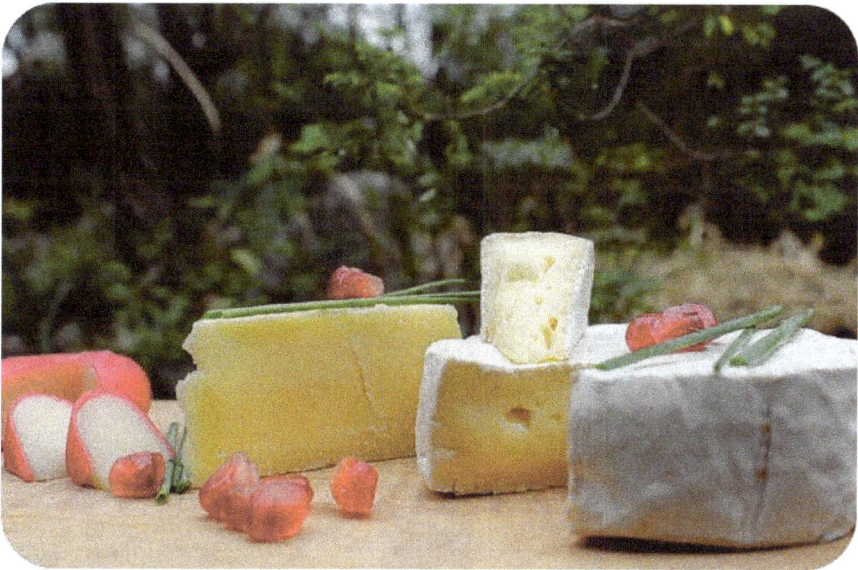

17. What should I do with a moldy coffee maker or kettle?

Mold in a coffee maker or kettle can grow in water reservoirs or damp spots, especially if not dried properly.

- **Light Mold**: Empty the water, scrub all removable parts with hot, soapy water, then run a cycle with a 1:1 water-vinegar solution to clean the internal system. Rinse thoroughly with clean water (run 2-3 cycles), and dry completely. If there's no lingering smell, it's safe to use.

- **Heavy Mold or Odor**: If mold has grown in hard-to-reach areas (like internal tubes) or the smell persists after cleaning, it might be time to replace the appliance. Mold spores can contaminate your drinks and pose a health risk.

- **Prevention**: Empty and dry the reservoir after each use, and leave the lid open to air out. Run a vinegar cycle monthly to keep mold at bay.

18. Can I still use a moldy shower curtain?

Shower curtains, especially plastic or vinyl ones, are mold magnets in damp bathrooms.

- **Surface Mold**: Wash the curtain with hot water and a cup of vinegar (machine wash if the label allows, or scrub by hand). For stubborn spots, use a 3% hydrogen peroxide solution (apply, let sit for 5 minutes, then rinse). Rinse, hang to dry fully, and check for odor. If it's clean, you can keep using it.

- **Deep Mold or Fabric Curtains**: If the mold has penetrated a fabric liner or the smell won't go away, toss it. Mold can embed in woven materials, and spores might spread in the humid bathroom environment.

- **Pro Tip**: After showering, spread the curtain fully to dry, and use a bathroom fan to reduce humidity. Spray with a vinegar solution weekly to prevent mold growth.

19. Is it safe to keep a moldy houseplant or its pot?

Mold on houseplant soil or pots often comes from overwatering or poor drainage.

- **Soil Surface Mold**: Scrape off the top layer of soil (about an inch) and dispose of it. Let the soil dry out completely, then repot with fresh, well-draining soil if needed. The plant is usually fine if the mold hasn't reached the roots.

- **Mold on the Pot or Plant**: Wipe the pot with a 1:1 water-vinegar solution and dry thoroughly. If the plant itself (leaves or stems) is moldy, it might be too far gone—trim affected parts, but if it's widespread, consider discarding the plant to avoid spore spread.

- **Prevention**: Water plants only when the top inch of soil is dry, ensure pots have drainage holes, and place them in well-ventilated spots with indirect light.

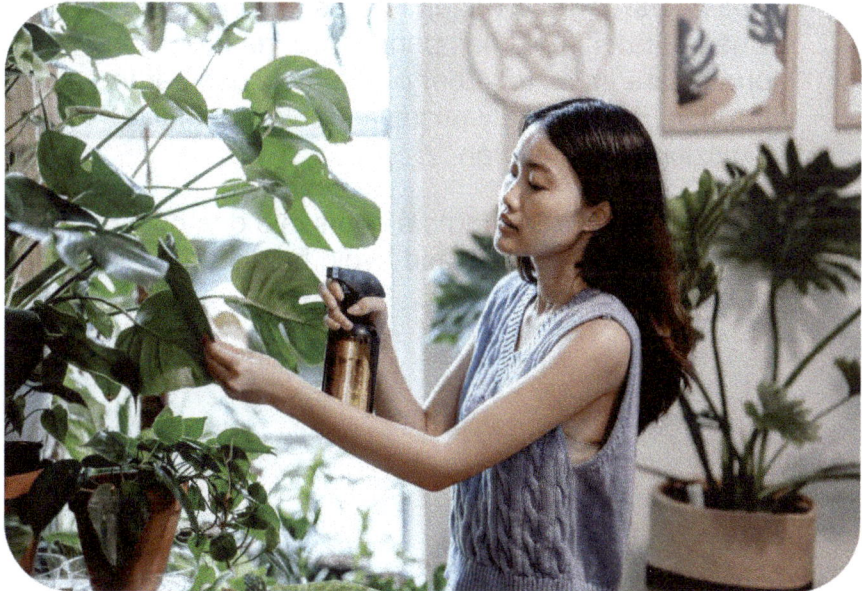

20. What do I do with a moldy photo album or framed picture?

Mold on photos or frames can be heartbreaking, but you might be able to save them.

- **Light Mold on Photos**: Isolate the album in a sealed plastic bag to contain spores. Gently brush off mold outdoors with a dry cloth (wear a mask). If the photo isn't damaged, wipe with a slightly damp cloth (1:1 water-vinegar mix), and air dry in sunlight. Scan the photo to preserve it digitally.

> **Myth:**
> You can eat fruit if you cut off the moldy part—it's still good.
>
> **Fact:**
> Soft fruits like berries are a lost cause—mold spreads deep; firm fruits like apples might be salvaged by cutting an inch around, but mycotoxins can linger.

- **Mold on Frames or Heavy Damage**: Wooden frames can be wiped with vinegar, but if mold has penetrated, replace them. If photos are stuck together or the mold has eaten through, they're likely unsalvageable—prioritize digitizing what you can.

- **Storage Tip**: Store photo albums in a dry, cool place with silica gel packets, and avoid humid areas like attics or basements.

Mold-Proof Living: Building or Buying a Mold-Resistant Home

Mold thrives in damp, poorly ventilated spaces, but the good news is that you can prevent it from the ground up—whether you're buying a home or building one from scratch. The materials you choose, the way you design the architecture, and the building practices you follow can make all the difference in keeping mold at bay. Think of your home as a fortress against mold: every decision, from the walls to the pipes, can either invite mold in or keep it out. Here's what to look for and prioritize to create a clean, mold-resistant living environment.

1. Choose Mold-Resistant Building Materials

Mold loves organic, porous materials that hold moisture, like untreated wood, drywall, or carpet. When buying or building, opt for materials that mold doesn't thrive on to reduce risk.

- **Ceramic Tiles:** Mold struggles to grow on non-porous surfaces like ceramic. Use ceramic tiles in high-moisture areas like bathrooms, kitchens, or basements. For example, a ceramic-tiled shower wall is far less likely to harbor mold than a drywall one, even if it gets wet daily.

- **Glass and Metal:** These are naturally mold-resistant because they don't absorb water. Glass shower doors or metal window frames (instead of wooden ones) can prevent mold in damp spots.

- **Mold-Resistant Drywall:** If you must use drywall, choose mold-resistant versions (often labeled "green board" or "purple board"). These are treated to resist moisture and are great for basements or laundry rooms.

- **Avoid Mold Magnets:** Skip untreated wood, paper-backed wallpaper, or thick carpets in humid areas. For instance, a shaggy carpet in a basement is a mold disaster waiting to happen—opt for a sealed concrete floor with a washable area rug instead.

- **Easy Example:** Imagine your kitchen counter—mold can grow in the grout of porous stone tiles if they're not sealed. Swap them for a solid ceramic or quartz countertop, which wipes clean and stays dry.

2. Embrace the Passive House Concept for Mold Prevention

Architecture is key to preventing mold, and the German Passive House concept, introduced over 30 years ago, is a game-changer. Passive Houses are designed to be ultra-energy-efficient while maintaining a clean, mold-free environment. Here's why this approach works:

- **Prevents Thermal Bridges and Condensation:** Thermal bridges are spots where heat escapes (like poorly insulated corners), causing cold spots where condensation forms—perfect for mold. Passive Houses use continuous insulation and airtight construction to eliminate these bridges. For example, a Passive House wall has no gaps, so the interior stays warm and dry, even in winter.

- **Forced Ventilation:** Passive Houses use mechanical ventilation systems with heat recovery to bring in fresh air while expelling humid, stale air. This keeps indoor humidity low (below 50%), which mold hates. Imagine a bathroom fan that runs automatically to whisk away shower steam—no more moldy grout!

- **Benefits of Passive Housing:**

    - **Mold Resistance:** By controlling humidity and preventing condensation, Passive Houses stop mold before it starts.

- Energy Savings: These homes use 5-10% more in upfront costs but save big on heating and cooling over time—often cutting energy bills by up to 90%. For example, a Passive House in a cold climate might need only a small heater, even in winter.

- Clean Air: The ventilation system filters out pollutants, ensuring a healthier indoor environment.

- Easy Concept: Think of a Passive House like a thermos—it keeps the inside temperature steady and dry, so mold can't find a foothold, while saving you money on energy.

3. Build to Keep Mold at Bay: Best Practices

Beyond materials and architecture, specific building practices can make your home a mold-free zone. Focus on keeping moisture out and air moving.

- **Insulate Ducts and Pipes:** Hot and cold water pipes, as well as A/C ducts, can collect condensation if not properly insulated, creating damp spots for mold. Wrap them in foam insulation to prevent moisture buildup. For example, an uninsulated A/C pipe in a humid attic can drip water onto the ceiling below, leading to mold growth—insulation stops this cold-sweat effect.

- **Slope the Landscape:** Ensure the ground around your home slopes away from the foundation to prevent water pooling near walls. A flat yard can trap water against your basement, seeping in and feeding mold. Aim for a 1-inch drop per foot for the first 6 feet away from the house.

- **Install Proper Ventilation:** Kitchens, bathrooms, and laundry rooms need exhaust fans vented to the outside (not the attic!) to remove humid air. For instance, cooking pasta without a fan can spike kitchen humidity, inviting mold—vent it out instead.

- **Use a Dehumidifier in Basements:** Basements are mold hotspots due to dampness. A dehumidifier keeps humidity below 50%. Pair this with sealing foundation cracks to stop water seepage.

- **Raise the Roof (Literally):** Design roofs with overhangs to direct rainwater away from walls. A short overhang lets water run down the siding, soaking it and encouraging mold—extend it at least 2 feet for protection.

- **Easy Example:** Picture a laundry room with an uninsulated dryer vent pipe. The warm, moist air cools inside the pipe, dripping water onto the floor—hello, mold! Insulate the pipe, and vent it outside, and the room stays dry.

4. What to Look for When Buying a Home

If you're buying rather than building, inspect the home with a mold-prevention mindset. Here's a checklist:

- **Check for Water Damage:** Look for stains on ceilings, walls, or floors—these signal past leaks that could harbor hidden mold. For example, a brown ring on a basement ceiling might mean a pipe leak upstairs, even if it's dry now.

- **Smell for Mustiness:** A musty odor, especially in basements or bathrooms, often means mold. Trust your nose—if it smells damp, investigate further.

- **Inspect Ventilation:** Ensure bathrooms and kitchens have working exhaust fans. Open cabinets under sinks to check for proper airflow—stuffy, damp spaces breed mold.

- **Look at Building Materials:** Favor homes with mold-resistant materials like ceramic tiles or metal framing over those with wall-to-wall carpeting or untreated wood. A home with hardwood floors is less mold-prone than one with carpet in every room.

- **Ask About Insulation:** Inquire if ducts, pipes, and the attic are insulated to prevent condensation. Uninsulated A/C pipes in a hot climate can drip and feed mold growth.

- **Hire a Mold Inspector:** If you're unsure, a professional mold inspection can test for hidden spores and moisture issues before you buy. It's a small cost to avoid a big problem.

- **Easy Example:** When touring a home, peek in the basement. If it's carpeted, smells musty, and has no dehumidifier, mold is likely lurking—pass on that house or plan for major updates.

5. Regional Climate Considerations and Old-World Wisdom

Mold risks vary by climate, so tailor your home design or inspection to your region. Combine this with time-tested, old-world practices—like using natural wind patterns—to enhance mold prevention naturally.

- **Humid Climates** (e.g., Southeastern U.S., Tropical Areas): High humidity fuels mold growth year-round. Prioritize dehumidifiers (aim for indoor humidity below 50%), extra ventilation (e.g., larger exhaust fans), and mold-resistant materials like ceramic or vinyl. For example, in Florida, a home without a dehumidifier in the basement is a mold disaster waiting to happen.

- **Cold, Wet Climates** (e.g., Pacific Northwest, Northern Europe): Rain and dampness increase the risk of water seepage. Focus on excellent waterproofing (e.g., sealed foundations, proper drainage), and insulate walls to prevent condensation from temperature swings. In Seattle, for instance, a home with poor roof overhangs might have constant siding moisture—mold's best friend.

- **Dry Climates** (e.g., Southwestern U.S., Deserts): Mold is less common but can still grow in poorly ventilated bathrooms or from plumbing leaks. Ensure good airflow in wet areas, and fix leaks immediately. In Arizona, a small, unnoticed drip under a sink can create a mold oasis in an otherwise dry home.

- **Old-World Wisdom:** Harness Natural Wind for Cross Breezes: For centuries, builders in windy regions—like the Mediterranean or Caribbean—designed homes to use the area's natural wind direction for cross ventilation. Position windows on opposite sides of the house to align with prevailing winds, creating a breeze that sweeps out humid air. For example, in a coastal area with steady east-west winds, place large windows on the east and west walls of your living room—open them, and the breeze will keep the space dry and fresh.

> **Myth:**
> Musty-smelling clothes are fine after a quick wash.
>
> **Fact:**
> That smell means mold's growing; a hot wash with vinegar might save them, but if it lingers or you see spots, the spores could be too deep—discard to avoid spreading.

- **Other Traditional Practices:**

  - **Elevate Homes on Stilts:** In flood-prone regions like Southeast Asia, traditional homes are built on stilts to keep them above damp ground, reducing moisture wicking into the structure. If you're in a flood zone, consider a raised foundation.

  - **Use Lime Plaster:** Old European homes often used lime plaster on walls, which is naturally mold-resistant due to its high pH and breathability—it lets moisture escape instead of trapping it like modern paints. Consider lime-based finishes for interior walls.

- ○ **Easy Example:** In a breezy coastal town, a home with windows aligned to catch the ocean breeze stays naturally dry, while a sealed-up house next door traps humidity and grows mold. Combine this with modern dehumidifiers for a double defense.

6. Why It's Worth the Effort

Investing in mold-resistant design might cost 5-10% more upfront (like the Passive House model), but the payoff is huge:

- **Health:** A mold-free home reduces risks of respiratory issues, allergies, or chronic illnesses like CIRS (Chronic Inflammatory Response Syndrome).

- **Savings:** Lower heating and cooling bills (thanks to Passive House efficiency) and fewer repair costs from water damage or mold remediation.

> **Myth:**
> Mold only grows in old, damp homes or basements.
>
> **Fact:**
> Mold thrives anywhere with moisture and organic material—even in new homes or behind drywall after a tiny leak.

- **Peace of Mind:** You'll rest easy knowing your home is a safe, clean sanctuary—not a breeding ground for toxic mold.

- **Real-World Win:** A family builds a Passive House with ceramic-tiled bathrooms, insulated pipes, a ventilation system, and windows aligned for cross breezes. They spend a bit more upfront but save thousands on energy bills over 10 years—and never deal with mold, even in a humid climate.

Free Resources to Track Your Recovery

Additional support for your journey with these free tools:

- **Mold Recovery Tracking Journal**: Prompts to reflect on wins, setbacks, and goals—keeps you motivated.

- **Weekly Mold Inspection Checklist:** A step-by-step guide to assess your home—checklist for leaks, humidity, and visible growth.

- **Monthly Symptom Progress Report:** A weekly log to monitor health changes, linking symptoms to exposure or interventions.

- **Home Maintenance Calendar for Mold Recovery:** A seasonal schedule for gutter cleaning, filter changes, and humidity checks.

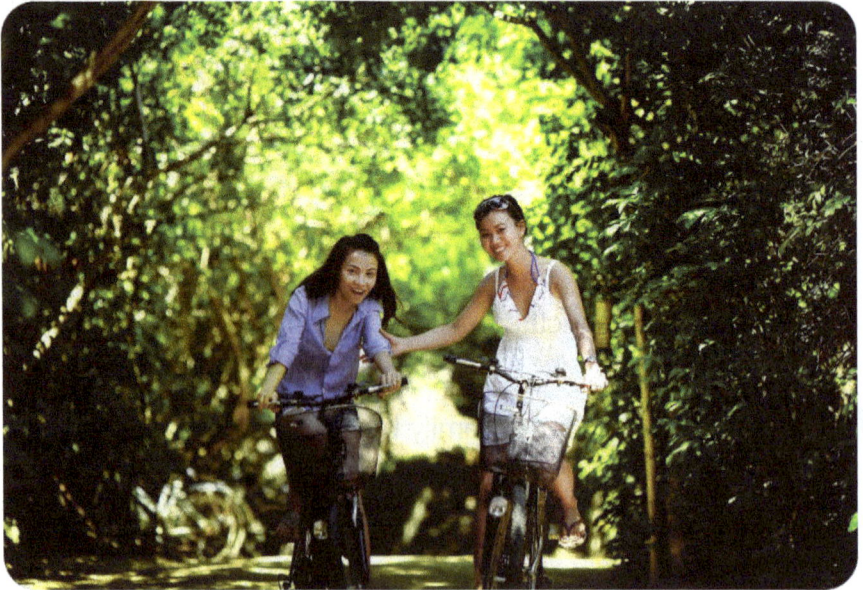

Mold Recovery Tracking Journal

Track your mold recovery daily to spot patterns and progress. Fill this out each morning—it helps you connect symptoms to fixes such as cleaning or detox, speeding your comeback!

Example Entry (Start Small)
March 20, 2025 | 8:00 AM | Rainy | 65% Humidity

- *Energy: 6 | Sleep: 5 | Hours: 7 | Headache: Yes | Dreams: No*

- *Symptoms: Fatigue (5), Brain Fog (5), Headache (4, forehead), Cough (2, morning), Sinus (3), Anxiety (3), Stuffy nose (2)*

- *Environment: Rain, Windows Open, Pet on Bed | Locations: Home, store | Outdoors: 1 hr | Pet Signs: No sneezing*

- *Interventions: Air Purifier (8 hr), Dehumidifier (4 hr), Cleaning (Peroxide, sink), Binders (Flax, 2 tbsp), Supplements (Vit C, 500 mg)*

- *Day Rating: 6 | Notes: Tea helped cough—basement still musty.*
  New? Start with date, energy, and one symptom—add more as you go!

Mold Recovery Tracking Journal

Daily Basics

Write date, time, weather—check humidity with a $10 meter. Knowing levels helps fight mold.

- Date: _____

- Time: _____

- Weather: _____ (e.g., rainy, sunny)

- Humidity (%): ___ (Tip: Aim for 30-50%)

Morning Check-In

Rate 1-10 (1=awful, 10=great)—tick quickly. Increased energy means progress!

- Energy Level: ___ (How awake do you feel?)

- Sleep Quality: ___ (How rested?)

- Hours Slept: ___

- Morning Headache: □ Yes □ No

- Dreams/Nightmares: □ Yes □ No

Symptoms (Rate 1-10: 1=worst, 10=best)

Check what applies—skip what doesn't. Notice what's slowing you down—patterns show you what to fix.

- Fatigue (__) □

- Brain Fog (__) □

- Headache (__) □ (Type/Location: _____)

- Cough (__) □ (□ Dry □ Productive □ Morning □ Night)

- Sinus Congestion (__) □

- Shortness of Breath (__) □

- Rash (__) □ (Location: _____)

- Itching (__) □

- Nausea (__) □

138

- Appetite Change □ Increased □ Decreased

- Joint Pain (__) □

- Anxiety (__) □

- Depression (__) □

- Memory Issues □ Yes □ No (Specify:
  _____)

- Dizziness □ Yes □ No

- Other: _____ (__)

Environment

Note surroundings—rain or pets matter. Notice triggers—humidity might be your clue.

- Conditions Today:

  - Rain/Humidity □

  - HVAC Use □

  - Windows Opened □

  - Other: _____ (e.g., pet on bed)

- Pet Signs: Sneezing □ Yes □ No | Other:
  _____

- Locations Visited: _____ (e.g., home, store)

- Time Outdoors: ___ hours

Interventions

List fixes—track what works. See if cleaning or detox lifts your day.

- Air Purifier (Run Time: ___ hours) ☐

- Dehumidifier (Run Time: ___ hours) ☐

- Cleaning (What/How: _____) ☐ (e.g., Peroxide on sink)

- Binders (Type/Dose: _____) ☐ (e.g., Flax, 2 tbsp)

- Supplements (Type/Dose: _____) ☐ (e.g., Vit C, 500 mg)

- Detox Methods (e.g., Lemon tea, Sauna): _____ ☐

Wrap-Up

Rate your day, jot down notes—keep it easy. Watch for wins— better days mean you're beating mold!

- Day Rating (1-10): ___ (1=rough, 10=awesome)

- Notes/Observations:

  _____

  (e.g., "Felt better after tea—basement still musty.")

Weekly Mold Inspection Checklist

Spot mold early with this quick weekly check—stop it before it grows! Takes 15-30 minutes—download the full 4-week version free at singingsoulbooks.com!

Example Entry (Start Simple)

Week of: March 20-26, 2025

- *Bathroom: Shower Corners ☐ | Under Sink ☐ | Toilet ☐ | Fan | Grout ☐*
  Notes: Grout dark—sprayed vinegar

- *Kitchen: Under Sink ☐ | Appliances ☐ | Dishwasher ☐ | Drip Pan ☐*
  Notes: Drip pan moldy—used peroxide

- *General: Sills ☐ | Vents ☐ | Plants ☐ | Basement ☐ | Attic ☐*
  Notes: Basement musty—dehumidifier on

- *Humidity: Bedroom 45% | Living Room 50% | Bathroom 60% | Basement 65%*

- *Tasks: HVAC ☐ | Dehumidifier ☐ | Purifier ☐ | Ventilation ☐*

- *Issues: Location: Basement | Description: Damp, musty | Action: Fan + peroxide*
  New? Start with one room and humidity—add more each week!

Weekly Mold Inspection Checklist
Week Basics

Write the week and grab a $10 hygrometer (e.g., Amazon)—keeping humidity at 30-50% beats mold fast!

- Week of: _____ (e.g., March 20-26, 2025)

Bathroom Check

Look for dampness or musty smells—mold loves wet spots!
Tick if clean, note fixes needed.

- Shower/Tub Corners □

- Under Sink □

- Around Toilet □

- Ventilation Fan □

- Grout Lines □

- Notes/Fixes: _____
  (e.g., "Grout dark—spray vinegar")

Kitchen Check

Check hidden zones—mold sneaks behind appliances! Tick if
clear, jot issues.

- Under Sink □

- Behind Appliances □

- Dishwasher Seal □

- Refrigerator Drip Pan □

- Notes/Fixes: _____
  (e.g., "Drip pan moldy—clean with peroxide")

General Areas Check

Scan common hideouts—dry areas win! Tick if good, note
trouble spots.

- Window Sills □

- AC Vents ☐
- Plant Pots ☐
- Basement Corners ☐
- Attic Inspection ☐
- Notes/Fixes: _____
  (e.g., "Basement musty—run dehumidifier")

Humidity Levels

Record with a hygrometer—high numbers mean act! Aim for 30-50% to stop mold.

- Room Readings (%):
  - Bedroom ___%
  - Living Room ___%
  - Bathroom ___%
  - Basement ___%

Maintenance Tasks

Tick what's done—these keep mold away! Small wins add up.

- HVAC Filter Change ☐
- Dehumidifier Emptied ☐
- Air Purifier Cleaned ☐
- Ventilation (Windows Open) ☐

Issues Found

Spot a problem? Write it down—fix it fast! Links to your action plan.

- Location: _____ (e.g., "Basement corner")
- Description: _____ (e.g., "Damp spot, musty")
- Action Taken: _____ (e.g., "Ran fan, sprayed peroxide")

Monthly Symptom Progress Report

Check your mold recovery monthly—see how far you've come and plan your next steps!

Example Entry (Start Simple!)
Month: March 2025

- *Health Metrics:*
    1. *Fatigue | 6 | 4*
    2. *Headaches | 5 | 3*
    3. *Brain Fog | 6 | 5*
    4. *Respiratory Issues | 3 | 2*
    5. *Skin Problems | 1 | 1*
    6. *Other: Sinus | 4 | 3*
    7. *Notes: Cough eased—still foggy some days.*

- **Treatment Compliance:**

    1. *Supplements: 80% (Vit C daily)*

    2. *Diet Protocol: 90% (Low sugar)*

    3. *Detox Methods: 70% (Flax most days)*

    4. *Environmental Changes: 100% (Dehumidifier on)*

    5. *Notes: Skipped flax some days—still helped.*

- **Environmental Improvements:**

    1. *Remediation □ | Equipment (UV-C lamp) □ | Adjustments (Lemon tea) □ | Maintenance (AC filter) □*

    2. *Notes: Basement dryer now—UV-C zaps books.*

- **Goals for Next Month:**

    1. *Run dehumidifier daily*

    2. *Stick to flax 100%*

    3. *Check attic for leaks*
       New? Start with 2 symptoms and 1 goal—add more next time!

Monthly Symptom Progress Report

Month Basics

Write the month—reflect on your daily and weekly logs to spot progress!

- Month: _____ (e.g., March 2025)

Health Metrics (1=worst/bad, 10=best/good)

Rate symptoms—lower severity means you're winning! Compare to last month or start.

- Symptom | Initial Severity (Start of Month) | Current Severity (End of Month)
    - Fatigue | ___ | ___
    - Headaches | ___ | ___
    - Brain Fog | ___ | ___
    - Respiratory Issues | ___ | ___
    - Skin Problems | ___ | ___
    - Other: _____ | ___ | ___
- Notes: _____ (e.g., "Cough eased—still foggy")

Treatment Compliance (%)

Estimate how often you stuck to fixes—consistency beats mold! Use daily logs to guess.

- Supplements ___% (e.g., "Vit C, 80%")
- Diet Protocol ___% (e.g., "Low sugar, 90%")
- Detox Methods ___% (e.g., "Flax daily, 70%")
- Environmental Changes ___% (e.g., "Dehumidifier, 100%")
- Notes: _____ (e.g., "Skipped flax some days")

Environmental Improvements

Tick what you did—small upgrades add up! Ties to your weekly checks.

- Remediation Progress Made ☐ (e.g., "Hired pros for basement")

- New Equipment Added ☐ (e.g., "Got UV-C lamp")

- Protocol Adjustments Implemented ☐ (e.g., "Added lemon tea")

- Routine Maintenance Completed ☐ (e.g., "Cleaned AC filter")

- Notes: _____ (e.g., "Basement dryer now")

Goals for Next Month

Set 3 targets—keep beating mold! Base on what's working or lagging.

1. _____ (e.g., "Run dehumidifier daily")

2. _____ (e.g., "Cut sugar more")

3. _____ (e.g., "Test attic air")

Home Maintenance Calendar for Mold Recovery

Keep your home mold-free with this seasonal checklist—small steps stop big problems!

Example Entry (Start Simple!)

Season: Spring (March-May 2025)

- **Indoor Maintenance:**

  - HVAC: Filters □ | Vents □ | Ducts □
    Notes: Vents dusty—wiped with vinegar

  - Humidity: Check | Dehumidifier □ | Fans □
    Notes: 60% bathroom—fan on

  - Plumbing: Pipes □ | Heater □ | Drains □
    Notes: Sink drip—fixed

- **Outdoor Maintenance:**

  - Gutters: Clean □ | Direct water □
    Notes: Downspout bent—adjusted

  - Roof: Roof □ | Vents □ | Cracks □
    Notes: Shingle loose—call roofer

- **Monthly Tasks:**

  - Visual | Humidity □ | Windows □ | Drip Pan □ |
    Fans □
    Notes: Drip pan mold—peroxide

- **Signs of Mold:**

  - Musty □ | Visible □ | Stains □ | Peeling □ | Warp □
    | Allergies □
    | Condensation □

  - Notes: Sneezing more—check basement
    New? Start with filters and humidity—add more
    next season!

Home Maintenance Calendar for Mold Recovery

Season Basics

Pick a season—use this to stay ahead of mold! Ties to your weekly checks.

- Season: _____ (e.g., Spring: March-May 2025)

Indoor Maintenance

Check these to stop mold inside—dry homes win! Tick when done.

- **HVAC System:**
    - Replace air filters (every 30-90 days) □
    - Clean vents/registers (e.g., vinegar wipe) □
    - Pro duct cleaning (if musty) □
- **Humidity Control:**
    - Check humidity weekly (30-50%) □
    - Test/clean dehumidifier □
    - Run bathroom/kitchen fans (30 min post-use) □
- **Plumbing:**
    - Inspect pipes/fixtures for leaks □
    - Check water heater for drips □
    - Clean drains (e.g., vinegar pour) □
- Notes/Fixes: _____ (e.g., "Fan loud—cleaned it")

Outdoor Maintenance

Keep water away outside—mold hates it! Tick when clear.

- **Gutters and Drainage:**
    - Clean gutters/downspouts ☐
    - Direct water 5 ft from foundation ☐
    - Check grading (slopes away) ☐
- **Roof and Exterior:**
    - Inspect roof (shingles/flashing) ☐
    - Check attic vents/screens ☐
    - Seal exterior cracks ☐
- **Landscaping (Summer/Fall):**
    - Trim plants (12 in. from house) ☐
    - Clear debris after storms ☐
- Notes/Fixes: _____
  (e.g., "Gutter clogged—cleared")

Monthly Tasks (Year-Round)

Do these every month—catch mold early! Small wins add up.

- Visual check (bathroom, kitchen, basement) ☐
- Humidity reading (adjust dehumidifier) ☐
- Window condensation check ☐
- Clean fridge drip pan ☐
- Test fans (bathroom/kitchen) ☐

- Notes/Fixes: _____
  (e.g., "Drip pan mold—peroxide")

Signs of Mold to Watch For

Spot these? Act fast—links to your action plan!

- Musty/earthy smells □

- Visible mold (even tiny) □

- Water stains (walls/ceilings) □

- Peeling paint/wallpaper □

- Warped wood □

- Worse allergies at home □

- Excess condensation □

- Notes/Actions: _____
  (e.g., "Musty basement—dehumidifier")

A Note of Encouragement

Whether you're just uncovering a mold issue or deep into your recovery, this book is your companion. You don't need to have all the answers today—what matters is starting. The journey may feel daunting, but it's also empowering. Each leak you fix, each breath of cleaner air, is a gift to your future self. Here's to your health, your healing, and the vibrant life awaiting you.

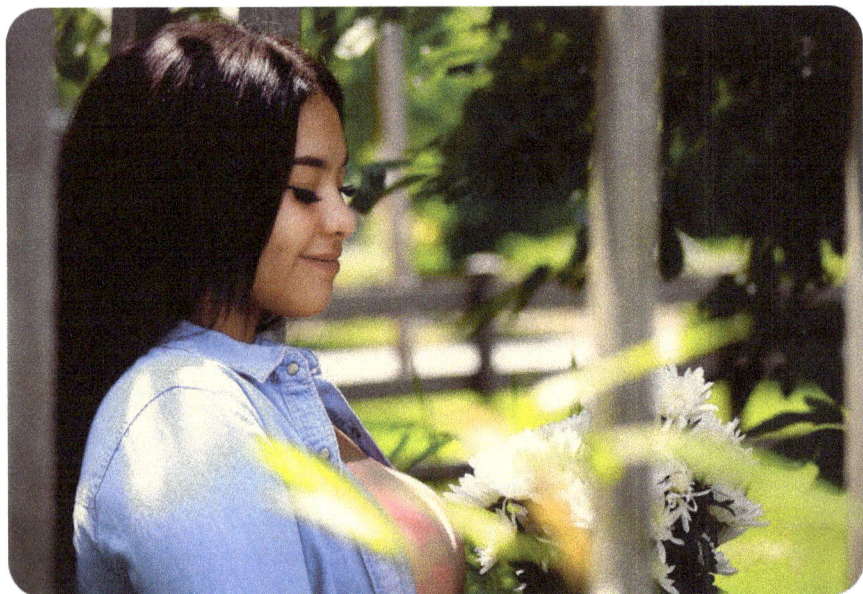

Glossary

- **BenzaRid:** A professional-grade mold killer, often lab-tested to eliminate 95-99.99% of mold. Commonly used in severe cases or by remediation experts.

- **Efficacy:** The ability of a method or product to kill or remove mold, typically measured as a percentage (e.g., 90% efficacy means it kills 90% of mold on contact).

- **Hydrogen Peroxide:** A liquid chemical (H_2O_2) that kills up to 90% of mold on contact. Works well on surfaces and porous materials, often used in DIY cleaning.

- **Mold Remediation:** The process of removing mold and repairing affected areas, usually done by professionals for large or toxic infestations.

- **Penetration:** How deeply a mold-killing method reaches into materials. High penetration (e.g., hydrogen peroxide) tackles hidden mold; low penetration (e.g., UV-C) only works on surfaces.

- **Surface Mold:** Mold growing on visible, non-porous areas like tile or glass. Easier to kill than mold in porous materials like wood or drywall.

- **Tea Tree Oil:** A natural essential oil with antifungal properties, killing 70-80% of mild surface mold. Often diluted in water for DIY use.

- **Thymol:** A natural compound derived from thyme, used in products like Benefect to kill nearly 99% of mold on surfaces. Eco-friendly alternative to chemicals.

- **UV-C:** A type of ultraviolet light that kills 99%+ of mold on exposed surfaces, according to EPA studies. Doesn't penetrate materials, so it's best for air or surface sanitizing.

- **Vinegar:** A common household acid (acetic acid) that kills 82% of surface mold. Affordable and safe for light mold on non-porous spots.

About the Author

Yvette Farkas is a holistic health consultant, bio-resonance expert, speaker, and author with over 25 years of clinical experience dedicated to transforming lives. Her comprehensive approach focuses on addressing the root causes of chronic conditions and empowering individuals to live their most authentic and vibrant life.

She specializes in supporting high-achieving individuals—particularly entrepreneurs, athletes, and executives—in overcoming perfectionism, self-doubt, loneliness, and anxiety.

With 30 years of martial arts training, Yvette brings unparalleled depth to her practice. Her approach artfully combines:

- Ancient healing techniques from Taoist and Ayurvedic medicine

- Acupuncture and nutrition strategies

- Energy healing and breathwork

- Laser therapy for improved healing

- A curated network of exceptional therapeutic professionals

Her 25 years of yoga practice further enriches her comprehensive wellness methodology, having empowered thousands to transform their lives through integrated mind-body approaches.

Yvette's expertise is deeply personal. Having navigated challenging life transitions—including a career-ending accident and battling debilitating health conditions like arthritis and chronic pain, she intimately understands the journey from rock bottom to renewal.

Her work has reached diverse audiences, including speaking at prestigious stages like MindValley University in Estonia, the Future You Summit in the UAE, and various Canadian and Hungarian organizations.

As the founder of Singing Soul Books, she has a unique approach to publishing that empowers authors to share their most meaningful narratives. Her literary portfolio spans diverse genres, from groundbreaking works on art and holistic health to her acclaimed children's book series, *Ethan and the Seven Chakras*, which ingeniously weaves coaching principles into captivating storytelling.

Yvette has earned national recognition with her books featured on CBC Radio and in The Globe and Mail. Her work has graced the shelves of the Art Gallery of Ontario (AGO) and secured a permanent place in the National Library of Canada—testaments to her impact on literary and cultural discourse.

At the heart of her work lies a profound mission: to inspire individuals to take control of their health and happiness, and live their most authentic vision.

Connect with Yvette

- **Website:** www.yvettefarkas.com

- **Bio-Resonance Services:** www.bioresonancescans.com

- **Publishing Company:** www.singingsoulbooks.com

- **LinkedIn:** www.linkedin.com/in/yvettefarkas

- **Email:** info@thesoulwhisperer.io